New Insights into Glaucoma

New Insights into Glaucoma

Guest Editors

Su-Ho Lim
Daniel Laroche

MDPI

Basel • Beijing • Wuhan • Barcelona • Belgrade • Novi Sad • Cluj • Manchester

Guest Editors
Su-Ho Lim
Department of Ophthalmology
Daegu Veterans Health Service Medical Center
Daegu
Republic of Korea

Daniel Laroche
Advanced Eyecare of New York
New York
USA

Editorial Office
MDPI AG
Grosspeteranlage 5
4052 Basel, Switzerland

This is a reprint of the Special Issue, published open access by the journal *Journal of Clinical Medicine* (ISSN 2077-0383), freely accessible at: https://www.mdpi.com/journal/jcm/special_issues/37J4096D9E.

For citation purposes, cite each article independently as indicated on the article page online and as indicated below:

Lastname, A.A.; Lastname, B.B. Article Title. *Journal Name* **Year**, *Volume Number*, Page Range.

ISBN 978-3-7258-7877-2 (Hbk)
ISBN 978-3-7258-7878-9 (PDF)
https://doi.org/10.3390/books978-3-7258-7878-9

Cover image courtesy of Daniel Laroche

Contents

About the Editors

Su-Ho Lim

Su-Ho Lim M.D. MSc. is Korean board-certified ophthalmologist and glaucoma specialist. He had worked as visiting Scholar @ Hamilton Glaucoma Center, UCSD Shiley Eye Institute, and Current Chairman, Director of the Department Ophthalmology, Daegu Veterans Health Service Medical Center, Daegu, South Korea. He graduated from Yeungnam University College of Medicine and Graduate School of College of Medicine (Ophthalmology). He finished his residency and clinical and research fellowship in Yeungnam Univ. Hospital. His main research interest includes diagnosis and surgical treatment of glaucoma, and minimally invasive glaucoma surgery. he published over 50 peer reviewed articles, contributed as first author or corresponding authors. He is currently academic editor for *Plos ONE* (Academic Editor), *BMC Ophthalmology* (EBM), *Journal of Ophthalmology* (Academic editor), *JCM* (Special Issue Guest Editor) and *Medicine* (Associate editor). He also has some patents regarding ophthalmic surgical instruments (glaucoma drainage device and strabismus hook). He has received several awards from various ophthalmologist societies (EVER, APGC, Korean Ophthalmological Society, and Korean Ophthalmologist Association, Sin-Mal Joint conference etc.) His office is in Daegu City, South Korea.

Daniel Laroche

Daniel Laroche is a board-certified glaucoma specialist, Director of Glaucoma Services and President of Advanced Eyecare of New York, and former Chair of the Ophthalmology Section of the National Medical Association. An internationally recognized ophthalmologist, he has performed thousands of glaucoma surgeries using advanced techniques including trabeculectomy, tube shunts, and microincisional glaucoma surgery (MIGS), and developed innovative procedures such as the Intrascleral Ciliary Sulcus Suprachoroidal Microtube and Retrobulbar Tube Shunt techniques to lower intraocular pressure. He created the Laroche Glaucoma Calculator to identify high-risk patients and prevent glaucoma through early intervention. Dr. Laroche earned his B.A. from NYU, M.D. with honors from Weill Cornell, completed residency at Howard University Hospital as Chief Resident, and a glaucoma fellowship at the New York Eye and Ear Infirmary. Board Certified, Ivy league trained, A Fellow of the American Academy of Ophthalmology, Co-founder of the Pan African Glaucoma Association and inaugural President, he has lectured internationally, received numerous awards for excellence and leadership, and remains deeply committed to advancing glaucoma care, equity, and medical education. His offices are in Southeast Queens and Harlem, New York City.

Journal of
Clinical Medicine

MDPI

Editorial

New Insights into Glaucoma—An Editorial Review on Broadening Risk Assessment, Refining Surgical Strategy, and Standardizing Clinical Practice

Su-Ho Lim [1,2,*,†] and Daniel Laroche [3,*,†]

1 Hamilton Glaucoma Center, Shiley Eye Institute, Viterbi Family Department of Ophthalmology, University of California San Diego, La Jolla, CA 92037, USA
2 Department of Ophthalmology, Daegu Veterans Health Service Medical Center, Daegu 42835, Republic of Korea
3 Advanced Eyecare of New York, New York, NY 10027, USA
* Correspondence: mdshlim@gmail.com (S.-H.L.); dlarochemd@aol.com (D.L.); Tel.: +82-53-630-7572 (S.-H.L.); +1-212-663-0473 (D.L.)
† These authors contributed equally to this work.

Glaucoma remains a major leading cause of irreversible blindness worldwide, with disease progression influenced by complex interactions, such as intraocular pressure (IOP), optic nerve head structure, vascular factors, multiple systemic diseases, and long-term treatment tolerability [1,2]. While lowering IOP remains the only proven strategy to slow disease progression, effective glaucoma care in practice is affected by various factors including accurate IOP measurement, treatment adherence, the management of coexisting ocular diseases, the appropriate selection of surgical options, and postoperative management [1,2]. In this context, this Special Issue of *Journal of Clinical Medicine*, "New Insights into Glaucoma" brings together ten studies that address these challenges across diagnostics, medical therapy, and surgery, offering pragmatic, clinically relevant evidence to inform and guide everyday decision-making.

1. Introduction

Glaucoma is a progressive optic neuropathy with highly variable clinical trajectories, even among patients with similar IOP levels and structural damage [1,2]. Large clinical trials and population-based studies have clarified the advantage of IOP reduction and identified risk factors including systemic, vascular, and treatment-related elements beyond IOP control alone [1,3,4]. The contributions in this Special Issue build on this foundation by highlighting how the measurement context, ocular surface health, affordability, surgical technique, lens extraction, affordable microinvasive glaucoma surgery, and systemic comorbidity can meaningfully influence outcomes over a patient's lifetime.

2. Measurement Matters: IOP as a Contextualized Parameter

IOP remains the cornerstone of glaucoma management; however, its interpretation is highly dependent on measurement conditions [2–4]. In routine clinical practice, IOP is frequently measured after visual field testing without considering the potential short-term physiological effects. Jang et al. (Special Issue) directly addressed this issue by demonstrating that automated visual field testing is associated with measurable changes in IOP when comparing pre- and post-visual field test measurements (DOI: 10.3390/jcm14186356). This finding is consistent with previous reports showing that perimetric testing itself can influence short-term IOP behavior [5] and has clear practical implications.

Measurement challenges are even more pronounced in pediatric glaucoma and eyes with anterior segment abnormalities. Studer et al. (Special Issue) compared Goldmann applanation tonometry, iCare PRO, and Tono-Pen measurements under general anesthesia in young children (DOI: 10.3390/jcm14103338). Their results highlight device-dependent differences that may affect longitudinal assessments, reinforcing the need for consistency in tonometry modalities and cautious interpretation of absolute IOP values in pediatric care.

3. Glaucoma Medication, Ocular Surface Health, and Sustainability

Long-term glaucoma medical therapy remains central to glaucoma care. However, its effectiveness is limited by ocular surface toxicity and poor adherence [6]. Preservatives such as benzalkonium chloride have been shown to induce inflammation, discomfort, and reduced quality of life, which in turn compromise treatment persistence and surgical readiness [1,6].

In this context, Kim et al. (Special Issue) conducted a randomized clinical trial to compare preserved and preservative-free fixed combinations of brimonidine and timolol (DOI: 10.3390/jcm14051587). Although the IOP-lowering efficacy was comparable, the preservative-free formulation demonstrated superior ocular surface outcomes and improved tolerability compared with the preservative-containing formulation in their study. Clinically, this study supports a shift toward treatment strategies that prioritize long-term sustainability over short-term pressure reduction alone, while also reminding us of the importance of surgery in reducing medication burden and the potential lifelong side effects associated with chronic topical therapy

4. Surgical Accessibility and Equity: Low-Cost but Effective Options

As the global burden of glaucoma has increased, disparities in access to surgical care have become increasingly evident. Calderon and Laroche et al. (Special Issue) addressed this challenge by evaluating a low-cost surgical approach, the Sinskey hook goniotomy combined with cataract surgery, in Black and Afro-Latino patients with glaucoma (DOI: 10.3390/jcm14103266). At one year postoperatively, clinically meaningful IOP lowering and a significant reduction in medication burden were achieved, with a high proportion of patients remaining medication-free. This study expands on previous work on angle-based minimally invasive glaucoma surgery by demonstrating that an effective glaucoma intervention does not always require expensive disposable devices [7,8]. Its inclusion in this Special Issue highlights its affordability as a legitimate dimension of surgical innovation and underscores the importance of aligning technique selection with population-specific needs, an especially important consideration for patients in resource-poor areas globally.

5. Surgical Outcomes: Techniques, Devices, and Preoperative Evaluation

Surgical success in glaucoma depends not only on the choice of procedures but also on tissue characteristics and perioperative management [9]. Several studies in this Special Issue illustrate how incremental refinements can improve outcomes. Yamazaki et al. (Special Issue) investigated whether preoperative exposure to prostaglandin analogs with differing potentials for prostaglandin-associated periorbitopathy (PAP) influences outcomes after trabeculectomy and Ahmed glaucoma valve implantation (DOI: 10.3390/jcm14196940). Their findings suggest that chronic topical glaucoma medication may affect periocular tissue response and relative surgical success, reinforcing the need to consider preoperative glaucoma medication history during surgical planning.

Device-based surgery is addressed in two complementary articles in this Special Issue. Kim et al. (Special Issue) present two-year outcomes of ab interno XEN45 gel stent implantation in open-angle glaucoma (DOI: 10.3390/jcm14134617), demonstrating sustained IOP reduction despite frequent early hypotony that generally resolved over time. In pseudoexfoliation glaucoma, Gehrke et al. (Special Issue) showed that temporary intraluminal nylon stenting during PRESERFLO MicroShunt implantation reduced early hypotony-related complications (DOI: 10.3390/jcm14176224). These studies highlight how postoperative safety can be improved through thoughtful modulation of aqueous outflow rather than wholesale changes in surgical strategy. In addition, a long-term perspective is essential. Fiore et al. (Special Issue) report five-year outcomes of deep sclerectomy in pseudoexfoliation versus primary open-angle glaucoma (DOI: 10.3390/jcm13237434), providing valuable diagnosis-specific data that inform patient counseling and long-term follow-up strategies.

6. Systemic and Sensory Dimensions of Glaucoma

Growing evidence supports a broader view of glaucoma as a condition influenced by systemic vascular and cardiometabolic factors rather than an isolated ocular disorder [1–4]. In this context, Lee and Seo et al. (Special Issue) employed a two-sample Mendelian randomization approach to investigate the relationship between atrial fibrillation/flutter and primary open-angle glaucoma (DOI: 10.3390/jcm13247670). Using genetic variants as instrumental variables, this study minimized the residual confounding and reverse causation inherent in conventional observational analyses and provided evidence supporting a potential causal association between atrial fibrillation/flutter and glaucoma. These findings extend previous epidemiological observations and underscore the clinical relevance of cardiovascular risk profiling and interdisciplinary collaboration for glaucoma care, while highlighting the importance of reinforcing healthy diet and exercise habits in our patients to maintain optimal cardiovascular health.

Beyond vascular comorbidity, Meliante et al. (Special Issue) explored the relationship between asymmetric glaucoma and ipsilateral hearing impairment (DOI: 10.3390/jcm13216501). Although exploratory, their findings raise clinically relevant questions regarding multisensory dysfunction and quality-of-life considerations, particularly in patients with unilateral or asymmetric diseases.

7. Concluding Perspective

The studies featured in this Special Issue collectively advance our understanding of glaucoma as a multifactorial disease influenced by ocular, systemic, and socioeconomic variables. Together, they emphasize that individualized care grounded in context-specific measurement, ocular surface preservation, surgical precision, and affordability can deliver sustained benefits over a patient's lifetime. By exploring innovations such as affordable microinvasive glaucoma surgery, combined with lens extraction, these contributions demonstrate that surgical success need not depend on costly instrumentation but rather on thoughtful adaptation to clinical contexts and patient needs, particularly in resource-limited regions.

Equally important, the findings underscore that comprehensive glaucoma management extends well beyond IOP reduction. The integration of systemic risk assessment, cardiovascular health promotion through diet and exercise, and a reduction in medication-related burden through timely surgical intervention represent a truly multidisciplinary approach. As this body of work shows, sustainable glaucoma care in the modern era relies on aligning technological innovation, clinical insights, and global health equity to secure meaningful, lifelong outcomes for patients across diverse populations. By integrating estab-

 https://doi.org/10.3390/jcm15031213

lished evidence from prior publications, this Special Issue offers personalized, long-lasting, and equitable clinically relevant insights into glaucoma management.

Author Contributions: Conceptualization, S.-H.L. and D.L.; methodology, S.-H.L. and D.L.; validation, S.-H.L. and D.L.; data curation, S.-H.L. and D.L.; writing—original draft preparation, S.-H.L.; writing—review and editing, S.-H.L. and D.L.; supervision, S.-H.L. and D.L.; project administration, S.-H.L. and D.L. All authors have read and agreed to the published version of the manuscript.

Funding: This research received no external funding.

Acknowledgments: The authors acknowledge the use of Paperpal Preflight (Paperpal, Cactus Communications) for assistance with English language editing. The scientific content and interpretations are the sole responsibility of the authors.

Conflicts of Interest: The authors declare no conflicts of interest.

Abbreviations

The following abbreviations are used in this manuscript:

IOP	Intraocular pressure

List of Contributions

1. Jang, W.J.; Chung, H.J.; Lee, M.W.; Kim, J.T.; Lim, H.-B.; Park, K.S. Effect of visual field test on intraocular pressure in glaucoma patients. *J. Clin. Med.* **2025**, *14*, 6356.
2. Studer, M.K.; Iliev, M.; Tappeiner, C.; Frueh, B.E.; Fraenkl, S.A. Comparison of intraocular pressure measurements with Perkins applanation tonometry, iCare PRO, and Tono-Pen in young children under general anesthesia with anterior segment abnormalities. *J. Clin. Med.* **2025**, *14*, 3338.
3. Kim, M.; Lee, C.-K.; Shin, J.; Kim, D.; Rho, S. Preserved versus preservative-free brimonidine/timolol fixed combination in patients with glaucoma: A randomized controlled trial. *J. Clin. Med.* **2025**, *14*, 1587.
4. Calderon, I.; Laroche, D. Affordable Sinskey hook goniotomy combined with cataract surgery in Black and Afro-Latino patients diagnosed with glaucoma: Retrospective real-world one-year results. *J. Clin. Med.* **2025**, *14*, 3266.
5. Yamazaki, I.; Kimura, M.; Sakamoto, R.; Kawai, Y.; Tsukamura, T.; Morita, H.; Kato, A.; Ozeki, H.; Nozaki, M.; Yasukawa, T. Preoperative prostaglandin analogues with high versus low prostaglandin-associated periorbitopathy–inducing potential and outcomes of trabeculectomy and Ahmed glaucoma valve implantation. *J. Clin. Med.* **2025**, *14*, 6940.
6. Kim, D.; Kim, M.; Lee, M.; Rho, S. Ab interno XEN45 gel stent implantation in open-angle glaucoma: Two-year outcomes. *J. Clin. Med.* **2025**, *14*, 4617.
7. Gehrke, M.; Keidel, L.F.; Buhl, L.; Priglinger, S.G.; Mackert, M.J. Early outcomes of intraluminal 10-0 nylon stenting during PRESERFLO™ MicroShunt implantation in pseudoexfoliation glaucoma. *J. Clin. Med.* **2025**, *14*, 6224.
8. Fiore, C.; Shang, X.; Lincke, J.-B.; Häner, N.U.; Zinkernagel, M.S.; Unterlauft, J.D. Five-year outcomes of deep sclerectomy in pseudoexfoliation glaucoma compared with primary open-angle glaucoma. *J. Clin. Med.* **2024**, *13*, 7434.
9. Lee, Y.; Seo, J.H. Potential causal association between atrial fibrillation/flutter and primary open-angle glaucoma: A two-sample Mendelian randomization study. *J. Clin. Med.* **2024**, *13*, 7670.
10. Meliante, L.A.; Coco, G.; Francavilla, B.; Bianchi, M.; Velletrani, G.; Di Girolamo, S.; Manni, G. Asymmetric glaucoma and ipsilateral hearing impairment. *J. Clin. Med.* **2024**, *13*, 6501.

https://doi.org/10.3390/jcm15031213

References

1. Gedde, S.J.; Vinod, K.; Wright, M.M.; Muir, K.W.; Lind, J.T.; Chen, P.P.; Li, T.; Mansberger, S.L. Primary Open-Angle Glaucoma Preferred Practice Pattern(R). *Ophthalmology* **2021**, *128*, P71–P150. [CrossRef] [PubMed]
2. Weinreb, R.N.; Aung, T.; Medeiros, F.A. The pathophysiology and treatment of glaucoma: A review. *JAMA* **2014**, *311*, 1901–1911. [CrossRef] [PubMed]
3. Meier-Gibbons, F.; Toteberg-Harms, M. Follow-up studies of the classical landmark studies in Glaucoma. *Curr. Opin. Ophthalmol.* **2023**, *34*, 116–122. [CrossRef] [PubMed]
4. Wishart, P.K. Interpretation of the glaucoma "landmark studies". *Br. J. Ophthalmol.* **2009**, *93*, 561–562. [CrossRef] [PubMed]
5. Li, M.; Zheng, B.; Wang, Q.; Sun, X. Impact of Visual Field Testing on Intraocular Pressure Change Trends in Healthy People and Glaucoma Patients. *J. Ophthalmol.* **2020**, *2020*, 7936205. [CrossRef] [PubMed]
6. Kim, D.W.; Seo, J.H.; Lim, S.H. Evaluation of ocular surface disease in elderly patients with glaucoma: Expression of matrix metalloproteinase-9 in tears. *Eye* **2021**, *35*, 892–900. [CrossRef] [PubMed]
7. Galvez-Olortegui, J.; Burgueno-Montanes, C.; Silva-Ocas, I.; Bernales-Urbina, S.; Galvez-Olortegui, T. Minimally Invasive Glaucoma Surgery (MIGS) recommendations in Clinical Practice Guidelines for open angle glaucoma and MIGS procedures: A scoping review. *Eur. J. Ophthalmol.* **2025**, *35*, 602–610. [CrossRef] [PubMed]
8. Lavia, C.; Dallorto, L.; Maule, M.; Ceccarelli, M.; Fea, A.M. Minimally-invasive glaucoma surgeries (MIGS) for open angle glaucoma: A systematic review and meta-analysis. *PLoS ONE* **2017**, *12*, e0183142. [CrossRef] [PubMed]
9. Gedde, S.J.; Feuer, W.J.; Lim, K.S.; Barton, K.; Goyal, S.; Ahmed, I.I.; Brandt, J.D.; Primary Tube Versus Trabeculectomy Study, G. Treatment Outcomes in the Primary Tube Versus Trabeculectomy Study after 5 Years of Follow-up. *Ophthalmology* **2022**, *129*, 1344–1356. [CrossRef] [PubMed]

https://doi.org/10.3390/jcm15031213

Journal of
Clinical Medicine

MDPI

Article

The Effect of Preoperative Use of High- vs. Low-PAP-Inducing-Potential FP Agonists on the Surgical Outcomes of Trabeculectomy and AGV Implantation

Iyo Yamazaki [1], Masayo Kimura [1,*,†], Risaki Sakamoto [1], Yukiko Kawai [1], Tomomi Tsukamura [1], Hiroshi Morita [1], Aki Kato [1], Hironori Ozeki [2], Miho Nozaki [1] and Tsutomu Yasukawa [1]

1 Department of Ophthalmology and Visual Science, Nagoya City University Graduate School of Medical Sciences, Nagoya 467-8601, Aichi, Japan; 14ymym.17@gmail.com (I.Y.); risakit13@gmail.com (R.S.); ykawai.medical@gmail.com (Y.K.); tomo.jk0629@gmail.com (T.T.); hiroshi1966morita@au.com (H.M.); akikato@cjimc-hp.jp (A.K.); miho.nozaki@gmail.com (M.N.); yasukawa@med.nagoya-cu.ac.jp (T.Y.)

2 Ozeki Eye Clinic, Ama-Gun 497-0050, Aichi, Japan; ozeki@dc5.so-net.ne.jp

* Correspondence: kimuram030301@yahoo.co.jp; Tel.: +81-52-721-7171

† Current address: Department of Ophthalmology, Nagoya City University East Medical Center, Nagoya 464-8547, Aichi, Japan.

Abstract: Background: Prostanoid FP receptor agonists (FP agonists) are widely used as first-line therapies for glaucoma but differ in their potential to induce prostaglandin-associated periorbitopathy (PAP), which may affect surgical outcomes. While several studies have reported an association between PAP and trabeculectomy failure, the impact of these agents on tube shunt procedures such as Ahmed glaucoma valve (AGV) implantation is not well established. **Methods**: We retrospectively analyzed 298 eyes of 221 patients who underwent trabeculectomy (n = 162) or AGV implantation (n = 136) between 2018 and 2023. The eyes were stratified by preoperative FP agonist use into the high-PAP-inducing-potential (bimatoprost or travoprost) and low-PAP-inducing-potential (latanoprost or tafluprost) groups. The primary outcome was the cumulative 2-year surgical survival rate under three intraocular pressure (IOP)-based definitions. **Results**: In the trabeculectomy group, the high-PAP-potential group had significantly lower 2-year survival rates than the low-PAP-potential group under all definitions. Cox proportional hazards analysis identified use of a high-PAP-potential FP agonist as a significant risk factor for surgical failure. In the AGV group, a difference between groups was seen only under the most lenient definition, with no differences under stricter criteria. **Conclusions**: The preoperative use of high-PAP-potential FP agonists is associated with poorer outcomes after trabeculectomy. Although the effect on AGV implantation appears limited, it may still influence early postoperative results. These findings underscore the need to consider PAP risk and medication history when selecting surgical procedures for glaucoma.

Keywords: glaucoma; trabeculectomy; Ahmed glaucoma valve implantation; prostanoid FP receptor agonist; prostaglandin-associated periorbitopathy

1. Introduction

Prostanoid FP receptor agonists (FP agonists), including bimatoprost, latanoprost, tafluprost, and travoprost, are widely used as first-line medications for glaucoma. However, these agents are known to induce various periorbital tissue changes collectively referred to as prostaglandin-associated periorbitopathy (PAP), including deepening of the upper-eyelid sulcus (DUES), ptosis, enophthalmos, and dermatochalasis [1]. Experimental studies have shown that these changes result from FP-receptor-mediated inhibition of adipogenesis and increased expression of type I collagen in orbital tissues, leading to periorbital tissue remodeling [2,3]. The incidence of PAP varies considerably depending on the specific agent. Bimatoprost has been associated with a high incidence of PAP (approximately 60–90%) [4–6], followed by travoprost (50–70%) [5,7], whereas latanoprost (6–41%) [5,6,8–10] and tafluprost (14–19%) [5,11,12] are associated with lower rates. These structural changes are thought to affect surgical outcomes, particularly in filtering procedures such as trabeculectomy, where successful bleb formation and maintenance are critical. For example, Miki et al. reported reduced trabeculectomy survival in regard to eyes treated with bimatoprost [13]. Moreover, the presence of DUES—more frequent with bimatoprost and travoprost—has been associated with poorer surgical outcomes [13]. A recent study using the Shimane University PAP (SU–PAP) Grading System further demonstrated that higher PAP severity is associated with lower surgical success [14].

In cases refractory to maximally tolerated glaucoma medications and conventional surgical interventions including trabeculectomy, tube shunt procedures are often considered [15]. Among these, Ahmed glaucoma valve (AGV) implantation is widely used, and its efficacy has been demonstrated in large clinical trials such as the Tube Versus Trabeculectomy (TVT) and Primary Tube Versus Trabeculectomy (PTVT) studies [16,17]. AGV implantation involves the insertion of a drainage tube and the creation of a bleb located approximately 8–10 mm posterior to the limbus. Due to its distinct anatomical configuration and different mechanism of aqueous outflow, AGV may be less affected by the structural changes associated with PAP. In fact, a recent study reported no significant associations between the severity of PAP and the surgical success rate following AGV implantation [18].

Given the anatomical and functional differences between trabeculectomy and AGV implantation, we aimed to investigate whether the preoperative use of FP agonists—particularly those with a high potential to induce PAP and DUES—differentially affects surgical outcomes. Based on previous reports [4–13], patients were stratified into two groups according to the agents used: the high-PAP/DUES-inducing-potential group (bimatoprost or travoprost) and the low-PAP/DUES-inducing potential group (latanoprost or tafluprost). Two-year outcomes were then analyzed separately for each procedure.

2. Materials and Methods

2.1. Study Design and Ethics

In this retrospective study, we reviewed the medical records of patients who underwent trabeculectomy and/or AGV implantation at Nagoya City University Hospital between January 2018 and September 2023. Only those with a postoperative follow-up period of at least one year were included in this study. The study was approved by the Ethics Committee of Nagoya City University (approval number: 60-23-0057) and registered with the UMIN Clinical Trials Registry (UMIN000057374).

2.2. Patients and Subgroups

The FP agonists used preoperatively included bimatoprost (0.03%) (Lumigan® Ophthalmic Solution; Senju Pharmaceutical Co., Ltd., Osaka, Japan), latanoprost (0.005%) (Xalatan® Eye Drops; Pfizer Inc., Tokyo, Japan), tafluprost (0.0015%) (Tapros® Ophthalmic Solution; Santen Pharmaceutical Co., Ltd., Osaka, Japan), and travoprost (0.004%) (Travatan Z® Ophthalmic Solution; Alcon Japan, Ltd., Tokyo, Japan). Eyes were categorized into two groups according to the type of FP agonist used: the high-PAP-potential group (bimatoprost or travoprost) and the low-PAP-potential group (latanoprost or tafluprost). Eyes were classified according to the type of FP agonist administered immediately prior to surgery, regardless of prior changes in medication or duration of use.

Trabeculectomy was performed using a standardized technique, which included a fornix-based conjunctival and Tenon's capsule incision; the creation of a 3.5 × 3.5 mm single- or double-layer scleral flap at the surgeon's discretion; the application of mitomycin C (0.4 mg/mL) for 3 min, followed by thorough irrigation with balanced salt solution; excision of the trabecular meshwork; peripheral iridectomy; and closure of the scleral flap and conjunctiva with 10-0 nylon sutures. Postoperative laser suture lysis was performed when necessary.

AGV implantation was performed using the Ahmed FP7 Glaucoma Valve (New World Medical, Rancho Cucamonga, CA, USA) in all cases. The procedure involved dissection of the conjunctiva and Tenon's capsule to accommodate the device, fixation of the endplate to the sclera 8–10 mm posterior to the limbus, the insertion of a tube into either the ciliary sulcus or vitreous cavity at the surgeon's discretion, coverage of the limbal portion of the tube with either a donor scleral patch or a half-thickness scleral flap, and closure of the conjunctiva.

2.3. Outcome Measurements

Outcome measures included intraocular pressure (IOP), use of anti-glaucomatous medications, and surgical survival rates. Surgical failure was defined as reoperation for glaucoma or loss of light perception. Reoperation included any additional glaucoma surgery (e.g., repeat trabeculectomy or tube shunt implantation) or laser procedures such as selective laser trabeculoplasty (SLT), conventional transscleral cyclophotocoagulation (CPC), and micropulse laser CPC (MP-CPC). Postoperative procedures such as bleb needling, laser suture lysis, or Yttrium–Aluminum–Garnet (YAG) laser use for relieving tube occlusion were not considered reoperations.

Surgical failure was defined based on IOP control, using three increasingly stringent criteria derived from the TVT and PTVT studies:

- Definition A: IOP > 21 mmHg or <20% reduction from baseline;
- Definition B: IOP > 17 mmHg or <20% reduction from baseline;
- Definition C: IOP > 14 mmHg.

All thresholds had to be met on two consecutive follow-up visits after 3 months. Eyes that required glaucoma reoperation or experienced loss of light perception were considered surgical failures regardless of IOP.

The primary outcome was the cumulative surgical survival rates stratified by the PAP-inducing potential of FP agonists used preoperatively: the high-PAP-potential group (bimatoprost or travoprost) versus the low-PAP-potential group (latanoprost or tafluprost).

IOP was measured using either a Goldmann applanation tonometer or an iCare rebound tonometer (iCare; Icare Finland Oy, Vantaa, Finland). IOP was evaluated at 3, 6, 12, 18, and 24 months postoperatively.

The anti-glaucomatous medication score was calculated as follows: 1 point per topical agent, 2 points for fixed-combination drops, and 1 point for oral carbonic anhydrase inhibitors, regardless of dosage.

2.4. Statistical Analysis

Statistical analyses were conducted using IBM SPSS Statistics version 30. Univariate comparisons were performed using the Mann–Whitney U test for continuous variables, including age, IOP, and medication score, and Pearson's χ^2 test for categorical variables, including gender, glaucoma type, history of prior glaucoma surgery, lens status (phakic or pseudophakic/intraocular lens), and preoperative FP agonist use. The Friedman test was used to analyze variance for nonparametric data with three or more time points, while the Wilcoxon signed-rank test was used for paired comparisons between two time points. Generalized estimating equations (GEEs) were used to analyze longitudinal data. Cumulative survival rates were calculated using the Kaplan–Meier method and compared using the log-rank test. Kaplan–Meier survival analyses were performed separately for Definitions A–C. Factors associated with the survival rate were analyzed using a Cox proportional hazards model. A p-value of <0.05 was considered statistically significant.

2.5. AI Tools Statement

ChatGPT (OpenAI, GPT-5) was used for English language editing of the manuscript. No AI tools were used for data analysis, content generation, or interpretation of results.

3. Results

3.1. Baseline Characteristics

A total of 298 eyes from 221 patients were analyzed. Of these, 133 patients (162 eyes) underwent trabeculectomy, and 110 patients (136 eyes) underwent AGV implantation (Table 1). The mean age was significantly higher in the AGV group (67.8 ± 12 years) than in the trabeculectomy group (65.0 ± 12 years). The mean preoperative IOP was also significantly higher in the AGV group (27.1 ± 11 mmHg) compared to that in the trabeculectomy group (21.0 ± 9.9 mmHg; $p < 0.001$, Mann–Whitney U test). In contrast, no significant difference was observed between the two groups in terms of the preoperative anti-glaucomatous medication score. The distribution of FP agonist use was also comparable between the groups. However, there were significant differences in the distribution of glaucoma types between the two groups, and the number of prior glaucoma surgeries was significantly higher in the AGV group.

Table 1. Baseline characteristics of patients who underwent trabeculectomy and Ahmed glaucoma valve implantation.

		TLE n = **162 Eyes**	**AGV** n = **136 Eyes**	p
Gender (n)	Male	88	88	0.069 [a]
	Female	74	48	
Age (years)		65.0 ± 12 (41~83)	67.8 ± 12 (31~90)	**0.002** [b]
Preoperative IOP (mmHg)		21.0 ± 9.9 (9.0~58)	27.1 ± 11 (10~70)	**<0.001** [b]
Preoperative anti-glaucomatous medication score		4.70 ± 1.2	4.68 ± 1.3	0.823 [b]
Preoperative prostanoid FP receptor agonist (eyes)				
bimatoprost		62	56	0.214 [a]
latanoprost		42	29	
tafluprost		39	23	
travoprost		13	18	
FP (-)		6	10	
Preoperative BCVA (logMAR)		0.174 ± 0.34 (−0.177~1.70)	0.446 ± 0.52 (−0.176~2.00)	**0.001** [b]
Preoperative MD (dB)		−15.5 ± 7.4 (−0.290~−32.7) (n = 129)	−13.7 ± 7.2 (−0.790~−32.9) (n = 77)	0.074 [b]
Lens status (eyes)	Phakic	98	69	**<0.001** [a]
	IOL	64	67	
Glaucoma type (eyes)	POAG/NTG	97	61	**<0.001** [a]
	PXG	21	16	
	Uveitis	29	15	
	NVG	3	14	
	others	12	30	
Prior glaucoma surgery (eyes)		65	85	**<0.001** [a]

Values are presented as means ± standard deviations or counts. Statistical comparisons were performed using the Mann–Whitney U test (continuous variables) and Pearson's χ^2 test (categorical variables). Bold values indicate statistical significance ($p < 0.05$). a: the Pearson's χ^2 test, b: the Mann–Whitney U test. AGV, Ahmed glaucoma valve; BCVA, best-corrected visual acuity; dB, decibels; IOP, intraocular pressure; IOL, intraocular lens; MAR, minimum angle of resolution; MD, mean deviation; NTG, normal tension glaucoma; NVG, neovascular glaucoma; PXG, pseudoexfoliation glaucoma; POAG, primary open-angle glaucoma; TLE, trabeculectomy.

3.2. Baseline Characteristics Stratified by the Type of FP Agonist Used: The High-PAP-Potential Group and the Low-PAP-Potential Group

Patients were divided into two subgroups based on the type of FP agonist used preoperatively: a high-PAP-potential group (bimatoprost or travoprost) and a low-PAP-potential group (latanoprost or tafluprost). In the trabeculectomy group, 75 and 81 eyes were in the high- and low-PAP-potential groups, respectively. In the AGV group, 74 and 52 eyes were in the high- and low-PAP-potential groups, respectively. The baseline characteristics of patients are summarized in Table 2.

Table 2. Baseline characteristics stratified by the PAP-inducing potential of prostanoid FP receptor agonists: high-PAP-potential group (bimatoprost or travoprost) and low-PAP-potential group (latanoprost or tafluprost).

	TLE			AGV		
	High-PAP-Potential n = 75 Eyes	**Low-PAP-Potential n = 81 Eyes**	p	**High-PAP-Potential n = 74 Eyes**	**Low-PAP-Potential n = 52 Eyes**	p
Glaucoma type (eyes)						
POAG	26	28		36	18	
NTG	19	23		2	3	
PXG	9	12	0.788 [a]	9	7	0.305 [a]
Uveitis	9	16		6	8	
NVG	3	0		7	5	
Others	9	2		14	11	
Preoperative IOP (mmHg)	22.0 ± 10	19.8 ± 9.9	0.102 [b]	25.8 ± 11	27.7 ± 10	0.105 [b]
Preoperative anti-glaucomatous medication score	5.07 ± 1.1	4.49 ± 1.1	**<0.001** [b]	4.93 ± 1.1	4.62 ± 1.1	0.079 [b]
Prior glaucoma surgery (eyes) *						
none	39	55		30	21	
SLT	20	15		26	14	
MP-CPC, CPC	1	1	0.258 [a]	5	4	0.695 [a]
TLO	11	11		8	10	
TLE	12	6		25	19	
Tube shunt	2	2		6	2	

Comparisons between groups were performed using the Mann–Whitney U test for continuous variables and the Pearson's χ^2 test for categorical variables. Bold values indicate statistical significance ($p < 0.05$). a: the Pearson's χ^2 test, b: Mann–Whitney test. *: Prior glaucoma surgery includes overlapping counts when different procedures were performed on the same eye. AGV, Ahmed glaucoma valve; CPC, continuous-wave cyclophotocoagulation; IOP, intraocular pressure; MP-CPC, micropulse laser cyclophotocoagulation; NTG, normal tension glaucoma; NVG, neovascular glaucoma; PAP, prostaglandin-associated periorbitopathy; PXG, pseudoexfoliation glaucoma; POAG, primary open angle glaucoma; SLT, selective laser trabeculoplasty; TLE, trabeculectomy; TLO, trabeculotomy.

There were no significant differences in the distribution of glaucoma types or the number of eyes that received prior glaucoma surgeries between the high- and low-PAP-potential groups in either surgical group. Preoperative IOP was also comparable between the high- and low-PAP-potential groups within each surgical group.

However, in the trabeculectomy group, the preoperative anti-glaucomatous medication scores differed significantly between the high- and low-PAP-potential groups, with a higher score in the high-PAP-potential group (5.07 ± 1.1) relative to the low-PAP-potential group (4.49 ± 1.1; $p < 0.001$, Mann–Whitney U test).

3.3. Intraocular Pressure

Changes in IOP stratified by the PAP-inducing potential of FP agonists are shown in Figure 1. In the trabeculectomy group, both the high-PAP-potential (bimatoprost or travoprost) and low-PAP-potential (latanoprost or tafluprost) groups showed significant postoperative reductions in IOP at all follow-up points compared to the baseline (Friedman test, all $p < 0.001$). In the low-PAP-potential group, the IOP reduction was significant at all time points, with $p = 0.001$ at 1.5 years and $p < 0.001$ at all other time points.

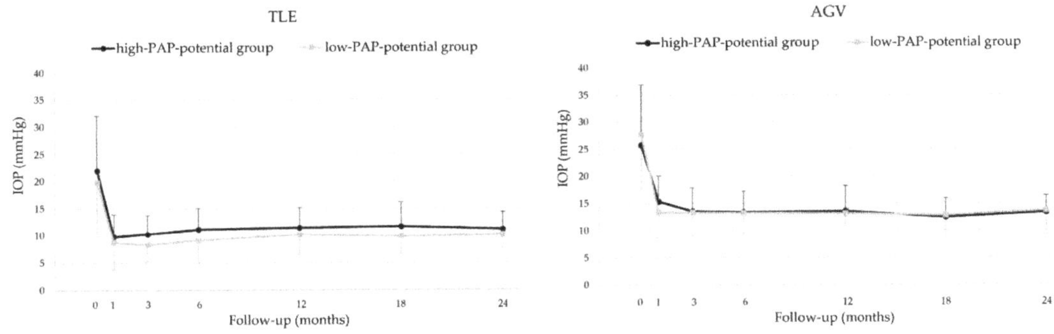

Figure 1. Postoperative intraocular pressure changes in groups stratified by the PAP-inducing potential of prostanoid FP receptor agonists. (**Left**): TLE group; (**Right**): AGV group. Eyes were divided into a high-PAP-potential group (bimatoprost or travoprost) and a low-PAP-potential group (latanoprost or tafluprost). In both surgical groups, IOP significantly decreased from the baseline at all follow-up points in both the high- and low-PAP-potential groups (Friedman test, $p \leq 0.001$ at all time points). No significant differences in postoperative IOP were observed between the high- and low-PAP-potential groups in either the TLE or AGV groups (GEE analysis, all $p > 0.4$). AGV, Ahmed glaucoma valve; GEE, generalized estimating equation; IOP, intraocular pressure; PAP, prostaglandin-associated periorbitopathy; TLE, trabeculectomy.

In the AGV group, both the high- and low-PAP-potential groups also exhibited significant postoperative IOP reductions at all time points compared to the baseline (Friedman test, all $p < 0.001$).

When comparing the postoperative IOP course between the high- and low-PAP-potential groups, no significant differences were observed in either the trabeculectomy or AGV groups (GEE analysis, all $p > 0.4$). There were no significant differences in preoperative or postoperative IOP between the high- and low-PAP-potential groups in either the trabeculectomy or AGV groups (Table 3).

Table 3. Comparison of preoperative and 24-month postoperative intraocular pressure between groups stratified by the PAP-inducing potential of FP receptor agonists.

		High-PAP-Potential Group	Low-PAP-Potential Group	p
TLE	Pre-surgery IOP (mmHg)	22.0 ± 10	19.8 ± 9.9	0.102
	24 months IOP (mmHg)	11.1 ± 3.2	10.2 ± 2.5	0.197
AGV	Pre-surgery IOP (mmHg)	25.8 ± 11	27.7 ± 10	0.105
	24 months IOP (mmHg)	13.3 ± 3.1	13.6 ± 4.4	0.985

Values are presented as means ± standard deviations. Comparisons were performed using the Mann–Whitney U test. High-PAP-potential group: bimatoprost or travoprost; low-PAP-potential group: latanoprost or tafluprost. AGV, Ahmed glaucoma valve; IOP, intraocular pressure; PAP, prostaglandin-associated periorbitopathy; TLE, trabeculectomy.

3.4. Anti-Glaucomatous Medication Scores

Anti-glaucomatous medication scores at baseline and at 24 months postoperatively were compared between the high-PAP-potential of FP agonists (bimatoprost or travoprost) and the low-PAP-potential of FP agonists (latanoprost or tafluprost) for both surgical procedures

(Figure 2). In the trabeculectomy group, both the high- and low-PAP-potential groups showed significant reductions in medication scores at 24 months compared to the baseline (Wilcoxon signed-rank test, both $p < 0.001$). The mean preoperative medication score was significantly higher in the high-PAP-potential group (5.07 ± 1.1) than in the low-PAP-potential group (4.49 ± 1.1; Mann–Whitney U test, $p < 0.001$). However, at 24 months postoperatively, there was no significant difference between the groups (Mann–Whitney U test, $p = 0.103$).

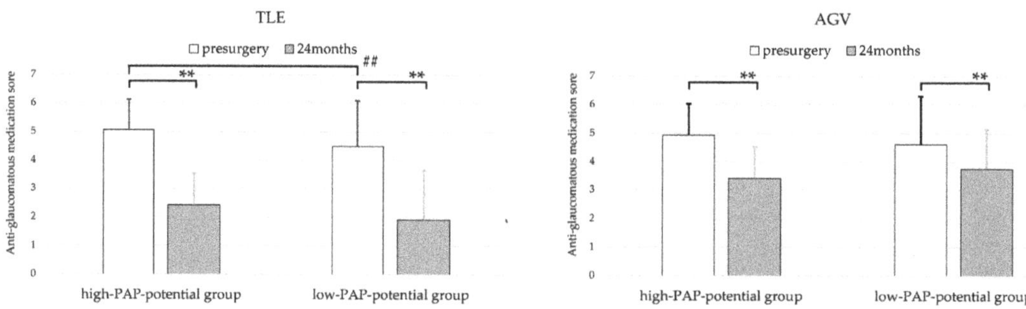

Figure 2. Preoperative (white bar) and 24-month postoperative (gray bar) anti-glaucomatous medication scores stratified by the PAP-inducing potential of prostanoid FP receptor agonists. (**Left**): TLE group; (**Right**): AGV group. ** $p < 0.01$ (Wilcoxon signed-rank test), ## $p < 0.01$ (Mann–Whitney U test). Eyes were divided into a high-PAP-potential group (bimatoprost or travoprost) and a low-PAP-potential group (latanoprost or tafluprost). In both surgical groups, anti-glaucomatous medication scores significantly reduced from the baseline at 24 months postoperatively (Wilcoxon signed-rank test: TLE, $p < 0.001$ for both the high- and low-PAP-potential groups; AGV, $p < 0.001$ for high-PAP-potential group and $p = 0.006$ for low-PAP-potential group). The mean preoperative medication score in the TLE group was significantly higher in the high-PAP-potential group than in the low-PAP-potential group (Mann–Whitney U test, $p < 0.001$). Error bars represent standard deviations. AGV, Ahmed glaucoma valve; PAP, prostaglandin-associated periorbitopathy; TLE, trabeculectomy.

In the AGV group, both the high- and low-PAP-potential groups also showed significant postoperative reductions in medication scores (Wilcoxon signed-rank test: high-PAP-potential group, $p < 0.001$; low-PAP-potential group, $p = 0.006$). There were no significant differences between the high- and low-PAP-potential groups in terms of either the preoperative scores (Mann–Whitney U test, $p = 0.079$) or the scores at 24 months (Mann–Whitney U test, $p = 0.460$).

3.5. Two-Year Cumulative Survival Rates and Factors Associated with Surgical Failure in Regard to Trabeculectomy

Two-year cumulative surgical survival rates following trabeculectomy were analyzed using Kaplan–Meier survival analysis and stratified by the PAP-inducing potential of FP agonists (Figure 3). The high-PAP-potential group (bimatoprost or travoprost) showed significantly lower survival rates than the low-PAP-potential group (latanoprost or tafluprost) under all three definitions (log-rank test): Definition A, $p = 0.034$; Definition B, $p = 0.034$; and Definition C, $p < 0.001$.

Factors associated with surgical failure pertaining to trabeculectomy were assessed using a Cox proportional hazards model for all three definitions (Table 4). The preoperative use of high-PAP-potential FP agonists was identified as a significant risk factor for surgical failure under all three definitions. Additionally, higher preoperative IOP was also a significant risk factor under Definition C.

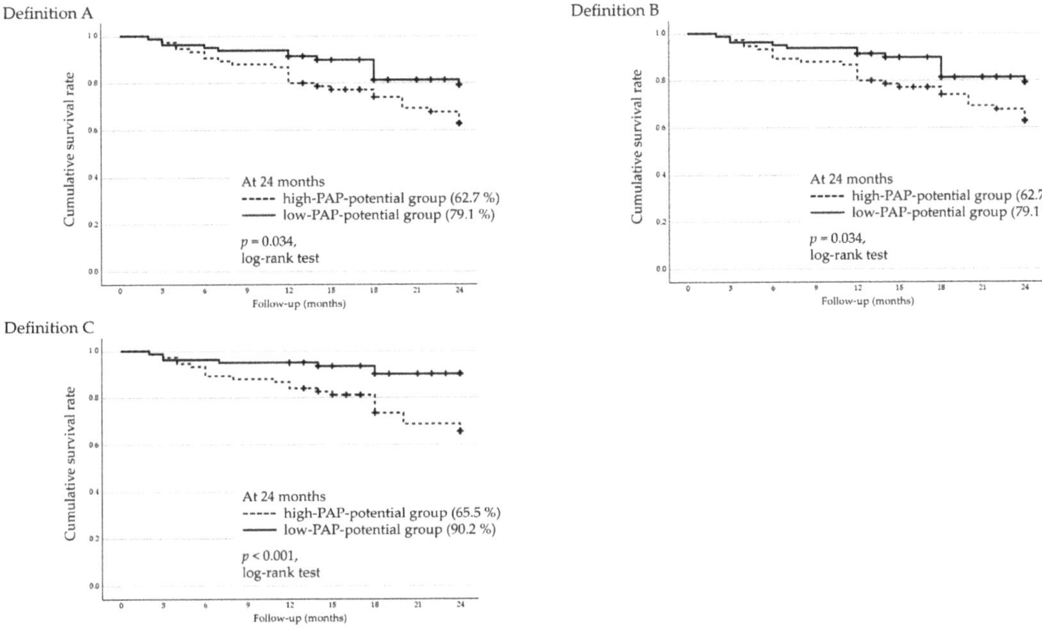

Figure 3. Kaplan–Meier survival curves for the trabeculectomy group stratified by the PAP-inducing potential of prostanoid FP receptor agonists. Eyes were divided into a high-PAP-potential group (bimatoprost or travoprost) and a low-PAP-potential group (latanoprost or tafluprost). Surgical failure was defined using three IOP–based criteria: Definition A, IOP > 21 mmHg or <20% reduction from the baseline; Definition B, IOP > 17 mmHg or <20% reduction; and Definition C, IOP > 14 mmHg. All criteria (Definitions (**A**)–(**C**)) were required to be met on two consecutive follow-up visits after 3 months postoperatively. The high-PAP-potential group showed significantly lower cumulative survival rates than the low-PAP-potential group under all three definitions (log-rank test). IOP, intraocular pressure; PAP, prostaglandin-associated periorbitopathy.

Table 4. Cox proportional hazards analysis of factors associated with surgical failure regarding trabeculectomy under Definitions A, B, and C.

	Definition A		**Definition B**		**Definition C**	
	Hazard Ratio (95% CI)	*p*	**Hazard Ratio (95% CI)**	*p*	**Hazard Ratio (95% CI)**	*p*
Glaucoma type	1.09 (0.926–1.28)	0.305	1.09 (0.926–1.28)	0.307	1.04 (0.881–1.23)	0.627
Prior glaucoma surgery (Yes/No)	0.588 (0.301–1.15)	0.121	0.589 (0.301–1.15)	0.121	0.495 (0.231–1.06)	0.071
Preoperative IOP (mmHg)	0.989 (0.953–1.03)	0.556	0.989 (0.953–1.03)	0.559	1.04 (1.01–1.07)	**0.005**
Preoperative anti-glaucomatous medication score	1.07 (0.802–1.41)	0.664	1.06 (0.801–1.41)	0.666	1.08 (0.782–1.50)	0.632
FP agent (latanoprost or tafluprost/ bimatoprost or travoprost)	0.473 (0.242–0.923)	**0.028**	0.473 (0.243–0.923)	**0.028**	0.271 (0.115–0.636)	**0.003**

Hazard ratios and 95% confidence intervals (CIs) are shown. Bold values indicate statistical significance ($p < 0.05$). IOP, intraocular pressure.

3.6. Two-Year Cumulative Survival Rates and Factors Associated with Surgical Failure in AGV Implantation

The two-year cumulative surgical survival rates following AGV implantation were analyzed using Kaplan–Meier survival analysis and stratified by the PAP-inducing potential of FP agonists (Figure 4). A significant difference was observed under Definition A, with the high-PAP-potential group (bimatoprost or travoprost) showing a lower survival rate than the low-PAP-potential group (latanoprost or tafluprost) (log-rank test, $p = 0.015$). However, no significant differences were found under Definitions B (log-rank test, $p = 0.112$) and C (log-rank test, $p = 0.680$).

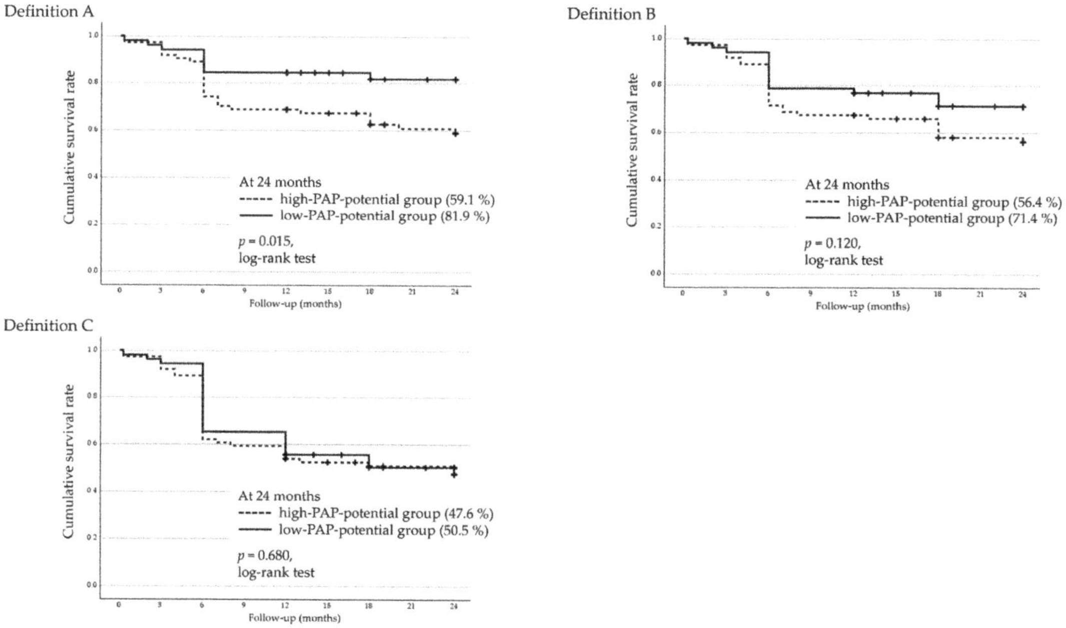

Figure 4. Kaplan–Meier survival curves for the AGV group stratified by the PAP-inducing potential of prostanoid FP receptor agonists. Eyes were divided into a high-PAP-potential group (bimatoprost or travoprost) and a low-PAP-potential group (latanoprost or tafluprost). Surgical failure was defined using three IOP–based criteria: Definition A, IOP > 21 mmHg or <20% reduction from the baseline; Definition B, IOP > 17 mmHg or <20% reduction; and Definition C, IOP > 14 mmHg. All criteria (Definitions (**A**)–(**C**)) were required to be satisfied on two consecutive follow-up visits after 3 months postoperatively. The high-PAP-potential group exhibited significantly lower cumulative survival rates than the low-PAP-potential group under Definition A (log-rank test, $p = 0.015$), whereas no significant differences were observed under Definitions B and C. AGV, Ahmed glaucoma valve; IOP, intraocular pressure; PAP, prostaglandin-associated periorbitopathy.

Factors associated with surgical failure in AGV implantation were assessed using a Cox proportional hazards model for all three definitions (Table 5). The preoperative use of high-PAP-potential FP agonists was a significant risk factor only under Definition A. Under Definition C, higher preoperative IOP was significantly associated with surgical failure.

Table 5. Cox proportional hazards analysis of factors associated with surgical failure in AGV implantation under Definitions A, B, and C.

	Definition A		Definition B		Definition C	
	Hazard Ratio (95% CI)	p	**Hazard Ratio (95% CI)**	p	**Hazard Ratio (95% CI)**	p
Glaucoma type	1.02 (0.895–1.17)	0.755	0.990 (0.877–1.12)	0.869	1.01 (0.906–1.11)	0.931
Prior glaucoma surgery (Yes/No)	0.592 (0.310–1.13)	0.111	0.625 (0.346–1.13)	0.120	0.729 (0.440–1.21)	0.220
Preoperative IOP (mmHg)	1.00 (0.967–1.03)	0.977	1.01 (0.983–1.04)	0.443	1.03 (1.00–1.05)	**0.026**
Preoperative anti-glaucomatous medication score	0.898 (0.686–1.18)	0.433	0.834 (0.652–1.07)	0.148	1.02 (0.815–1.27)	0.887
FP agent (latanoprost or tafluprost/ bimatoprost or travoprost)	0.402 (0.189–0.856)	**0.018**	0.597 (0.315–1.13)	0.120	0.834 (0.500–1.392)	0.487

Hazard ratios and 95% confidence intervals (CIs) are shown. Bold values indicate statistical significance ($p < 0.05$). IOP, intraocular pressure.

4. Discussion

FP agonists are widely used as first-line treatments for glaucoma, but they differ in their propensity to induce periorbital changes, such as PAP including DUES [1]. Bimatoprost and travoprost have been reported to promote eyelid stiffening and orbital fat atrophy by enhancing type I collagen expression and suppressing adipogenesis [2,3]. These histological changes underlie the development of PAP, which has been reported in 50–93% of patients treated with these agents [4–7]. In contrast, latanoprost and tafluprost are associated with a lower risk of such adverse effects. Although latanoprost also exhibits lipolytic and fibrotic activity [2,3], its limited accumulation in orbital tissues is thought to contribute to the lower reported incidence of DUES (6–41%) [5,6,8–10,19]. Tafluprost, a highly selective FP agonist with lower cytotoxicity and inflammatory potential [20,21], has been associated with low DUES rates of only 14–19% [5,11,12].

In this study, we stratified preoperative FP agonists into high-PAP-potential (bimatoprost and travoprost) and low-PAP-potential (latanoprost and tafluprost) categories based on their known propensity to cause PAP. We then compared the surgical outcomes of trabeculectomy and AGV implantation between these groups.

In the trabeculectomy group, the high-PAP-potential group exhibited significantly lower cumulative survival across all definitions of surgical failure. Cox proportional hazards analysis identified the preoperative use of high-PAP-potential FP agonists as a consistent predictor of surgical failure. Among the other tested factors, only higher preoperative IOP was significantly associated with surgical failure under Definition C, whereas glaucoma type, prior glaucoma surgery, and preoperative anti-glaucomatous medication score showed no significant associations. These findings suggest that PAP-associated changes—including eyelid stiffness, fibrosis, and fat atrophy—may compromise the formation and long-term viability of filtering blebs. Although this study did not include direct clinical imaging assessment of PAP or DUES, the observed outcome differences are consistent with previous reports highlighting the detrimental impact of PAP on trabeculectomy [13,14].

In the AGV group, a significant difference between the high- and low-PAP-potential groups was observed only under the lenient Definition A, while no significant differences were found under the stricter Definitions B and C. The Kaplan–Meier curves demonstrated a noticeable drop in survival rates around six months postoperatively across all groups.

This timing coincides with the known hypertensive phase, which occurs in 56–82% of eyes within 3 to 6 months after AGV surgery and is associated with worse long-term outcomes [22–24]. The early postoperative decline in survival rates may indicate that the hypertensive phase had a greater impact on surgical outcomes, particularly for eyes with pre-existing PAP-associated changes, which were more common in the high-PAP-potential group. Definition A, being more permissive in terms of IOP criteria, may have been more sensitive in capturing these early failures.

Long-term exposure to bimatoprost or travoprost may result in advanced periorbital fibrosis and fat atrophy, potentially contributing to fibrous encapsulation of the AGV endplate and unstable postoperative IOP control during the hypertensive phase. In contrast, eyes treated with low-PAP-potential agents (latanoprost or tafluprost) may have had less pre-existing fibrosis, enabling them to maintain acceptable IOP control under a more permissive failure definition. However, under stricter criteria, the results did not reach statistical significance (Definition B: HR = 0.597, 95% CI 0.315–1.13, $p = 0.120$; Definition C: HR = 0.834, 95% CI 0.500–1.392, $p = 0.487$). The lack of significance under Definition B was most likely due to the limited number of events in the AGV subgroup, whereas under Definition C, the stringent cutoff (>14 mmHg) markedly reduced discriminatory ability, with approximately half of the cases classified as failures regardless of medication history. Although this threshold may indeed be overly demanding for tube shunt procedures that generally aim for relatively higher target pressures, we adopted it in line with previous landmark studies, such as the TVT and PTVT trials [16,17], to ensure comparability with prior research. Among the other tested factors, only higher preoperative IOP was significantly associated with surgical failure under Definition C, whereas glaucoma type, prior glaucoma surgery, and preoperative anti-glaucomatous medication score showed no significant associations. Although postoperative medication scores decreased significantly after AGV implantation, the absolute magnitude of this reduction was modest (approximately one medication), and thus its clinical significance should be interpreted with caution. These observations suggest that, while the influence of PAP is less prominent in AGV implantation compared to trabeculectomy, it should still be considered, particularly in the early postoperative period and for patients with a history of high-PAP-potential FP agonist use.

In trabeculectomy, bleb morphology is influenced by anterior periorbital tissues, and the SU-PAP grading system may be useful for predicting surgical outcomes [14]. In contrast, AGV implantation results in bleb formation approximately 8–10 mm posterior to the limbus. This deeper and more posterior anatomical configuration likely reduces the mechanical influence of PAP-related changes such as eyelid stiffness or orbital fibrosis, and thus the effects of PAP on AGV outcomes may be minimal. Although Harano et al. found no association between SU-PAP grades and AGV outcomes [18], this may have been due to the system's reliance on external periorbital appearance, which may not fully reflect the condition of deeper orbital tissues surrounding the AGV bleb. Therefore, when evaluating indications for AGV and predicting surgical outcomes, a comprehensive assessment—including the severity of PAP and particularly the history of high-PAP-inducing FP agonist use—may be necessary.

This study has several limitations. First, as a retrospective study, direct clinical imaging assessment of PAP, including DUES, was not possible due to insufficient documentation in most medical records. Second, the classification into high- and low-PAP-potential groups was based solely on the final preoperative medication, without accounting for prior exposure, drug switching, or cumulative duration of use. Third, postoperative bleb morphology or anterior segment optical coherence tomography data were not available, which precluded analysis of their correlation with preoperative medication history. Fourth, because AGV is generally reserved for refractory cases, baseline disease severity and prior surgical history may have influenced the outcomes. Fifth, the relatively small sample size, particularly in the AGV group, may limit the applicability of our findings. Finally, as this is a single-center study, the results may not be fully generalizable to other populations or clinical settings.

5. Conclusions

This study demonstrates that preoperative use of high-PAP-inducing-potential agents was significantly associated with poorer surgical outcomes of trabeculectomy, while the impact was more limited in regard to AGV implantation. These findings underscore the importance of considering not only observable signs of PAP but also the patient's medication history when selecting a surgical approach for glaucoma. Future prospective studies with larger sample sizes, longer follow-up periods, and direct assessment of PAP including DUES are warranted to further elucidate these associations and support evidence-based surgical decision-making.

Author Contributions: Conceptualization, M.K. and M.N.; methodology, M.K.; software, I.Y. and M.K.; validation, I.Y., M.K., H.M., A.K. and T.Y.; formal analysis, I.Y. and M.K.; investigation, I.Y., Y.K., R.S. and H.O.; data curation, M.K., T.T., H.M., A.K. and T.Y.; writing—original draft preparation, I.Y.; writing—review and editing, M.K., A.K. and M.N.; visualization, M.K.; supervision, M.K., M.N. and T.Y.; project administration, M.K. and M.N. All authors have read and agreed to the published version of the manuscript.

Funding: This research was funded by a Grant-in-Aid for Young Scientists, Japan Society for the Promotion of Science, under grant number 23K15913 (M.K.); Grant-in-Aid for Scientific Research (B), Japan Society for the Promotion of Science, under grant number 23K24502 and 25K02795 (T.Y.); and the Nagoya Co-Creation Research Fund (M.N.).

Institutional Review Board Statement: This study was conducted in accordance with the Declaration of Helsinki and approved by the Institutional Review Board of Nagoya City University Graduate School of Medical Science (protocol code: 60-23-0057; date of first approval: 13 September 2023).

Informed Consent Statement: Patient consent was waived due to the retrospective observational nature of this study, but an explanatory document regarding the study was made publicly available. The document outlined (1) the purpose and methods of the study, (2) that patients may refuse at any time to allow their data to be used, (3) that patient privacy is protected, (4) that there are no conflicts of interest in the study, and (5) that the study was approved by an ethical review board.

Data Availability Statement: Researchers can contact Masayo Kimura, (kimuram030301@yahoo.co.jp), to obtain details of the protocol and results.

Acknowledgments: During the preparation of this manuscript, the authors used ChatGPT (OpenAI, GPT-5) for the purposes of English language editing. The authors also received professional English language editing support from MDPI Author Services. The authors have reviewed and edited the output and take full responsibility for the content of this publication.

Conflicts of Interest: The authors declare no conflicts of interest.

Abbreviations

The following abbreviations are used in this manuscript:

AGV	Ahmed glaucoma valve
ANOVA	analysis of variance
BCVA	best-corrected visual acuity
BGI	Baerveldt glaucoma implant
CI	confidence interval
CPC	cyclophotocoagulation
dB	decibels
DUES	deepening of upper-eyelid sulcus
GEE	Generalized estimating equation
IOL	intraocular lens
IOP	intraocular pressure
MAR	minimum angle of resolution
MD	mean deviation
MP-CPC	micropulse laser cyclophotocoagulation
NTG	normal tension glaucoma
NVG	neovascular glaucoma
PAP	prostaglandin-associated periorbitopathy
PXG	pseudoexfoliation glaucoma
POAG	primary open-angle glaucoma
PTVT	Primary Tube Versus Trabeculectomy
SLT	selective laser trabeculoplasty
SU	Shimane University
TLE	trabeculectomy
TLO	trabeculotomy
TVT	Tube Versus Trabeculectomy

References

1. Alm, A.; Grierson, I.; Shields, M.B. Side effects associated with prostaglandin analog therapy. *Surv. Ophthalmol.* **2008**, *53* (Suppl. 1), S93–S105. [CrossRef]
2. Taketani, Y.; Yamagishi, R.; Fujishiro, T.; Igarashi, M.; Sakata, R.; Aihara, M. Activation of the prostanoid FP receptor inhibits adipogenesis leading to deepening of the upper eyelid sulcus in prostaglandin-associated periorbitopathy. *Investig. Ophthalmol. Vis. Sci.* **2014**, *55*, 1269–1276. [CrossRef]
3. Itoh, K.; Ida, Y.; Ohguro, H.; Hikage, F. Prostaglandin F2α agonists induced enhancement in collagen1 expression is involved in the pathogenesis of the deepening of upper eyelid sulcus. *Sci. Rep.* **2021**, *11*, 9002. [CrossRef] [PubMed]
4. Aihara, M.; Shirato, S.; Sakata, R. Incidence of deepening of the upper eyelid sulcus after switching from latanoprost to bimatoprost. *Jpn. J. Ophthalmol.* **2011**, *55*, 600–604. [CrossRef] [PubMed]
5. Inoue, K.; Shiokawa, M.; Wakakura, M.; Tomita, G. Deepening of the upper eyelid sulcus caused by 5 types of prostaglandin analogs. *J. Glaucoma* **2013**, *22*, 626–631. [CrossRef] [PubMed]
6. Kucukevcilioglu, M.; Bayer, A.; Uysal, Y.; Altinsoy, H.I. Prostaglandin associated periorbitopathy in patients using bimatoprost, latanoprost and travoprost. *Clin. Exp. Ophthalmol.* **2014**, *42*, 126–131. [CrossRef]
7. Maruyama, K.; Shirato, S.; Tsuchisaka, A. Incidence of deepening of the upper eyelid sulcus after topical use of travoprost ophthalmic solution in Japanese. *J. Glaucoma* **2014**, *23*, 160–163. [CrossRef]
8. Sakata, R.; Shirato, S.; Miyata, K.; Aihara, M. Incidence of deepening of the upper eyelid sulcus in prostaglandin-associated periorbitopathy with a latanoprost ophthalmic solution. *Eye* **2014**, *28*, 1446–1451. [CrossRef]
9. Nakakura, S.; Yamamoto, M.; Terao, E.; Nagatomi, N.; Matsuo, N.; Fujisawa, Y.; Fujio, Y.; Tabuchi, H.; Kiuchi, Y. Prostaglandin-associated periorbitopathy in latanoprost users. *Clin. Ophthalmol.* **2014**, *30*, 51–56. [CrossRef]
10. Alm, A. Latanoprost in the treatment of glaucoma. *Clin. Ophthalmol.* **2014**, *26*, 1967–1985. [CrossRef]
11. Maruyama, K.; Tsuchisaka, A.; Sakamoto, J.; Shirato, S.; Goto, H. Incidence of deepening of upper eyelid sulcus after topical use of tafluprost ophthalmic solution in Japanese patients. *Clin. Ophthalmol.* **2013**, *7*, 1441–1446. [CrossRef] [PubMed]
12. Sakata, R.; Shirato, S.; Miyata, K.; Aihara, M. Incidence of deepening of the upper eyelid sulcus on treatment with a tafluprost ophthalmic solution. *Jpn. J. Ophthalmol.* **2014**, *58*, 212–217. [CrossRef] [PubMed]
13. Miki, T.; Naito, T.; Fujiwara, M.; Araki, R.; Kiyoi, R.; Shiode, Y.; Fujiwara, A.; Morizane, Y.; Shiraga, F. Effects of pre-surgical administration of prostaglandin analogs on the outcome of trabeculectomy. *PLoS ONE* **2017**, *12*, e0181550. [CrossRef] [PubMed]

14. Ishida, A.; Miki, T.; Naito, T.; Ichioka, S.; Takayanagi, Y.; Tanito, M. Surgical Results of Trabeculectomy among Groups Stratified by Prostaglandin-Associated Periorbitopathy Severity. *Ophthalmology* **2023**, *130*, 297–303. [CrossRef]
15. Kiuchi, Y.; Inoue, T.; Shoji, N.; Nakamura, M.; Tanito, M.; Glaucoma Guideline Preparation Committee, Japan Glaucoma Society. The Japan Glaucoma Society guidelines for glaucoma, 5th edition. *Jpn. J. Ophthalmol.* **2023**, *67*, 189–254. [CrossRef]
16. Gedde, S.J.; Schiffman, J.C.; Feuer, W.J.; Herndon, L.W.; Brandt, J.D.; Budenz, D.L.; Tube versus Trabeculectomy Study Group. Treatment outcomes in the Tube Versus Trabeculectomy (TVT) study after five years of follow-up. *Am. J. Ophthalmol.* **2012**, *153*, 789–803.e2. [CrossRef]
17. Gedde, S.J.; Feuer, W.J.; Lim, K.S.; Barton, K.; Goyal, S.; Ahmed, I.I.; Brandt, J.D.; Primary Tube Versus Trabeculectomy Study Group. Treatment Outcomes in the Primary Tube Versus Trabeculectomy Study after 5 Years of Follow-up. *Ophthalmology* **2022**, *129*, 1344–1356. [CrossRef]
18. Harano, A.; Ichioka, S.; Murakami, K.; Iida, M.; Tanito, M. The Severity of Prostaglandin-Associated Periorbitopathy Did Not Affect the Surgical Effectiveness of the Ahmed Glaucoma Valve. *J. Clin. Med.* **2024**, *14*, 42. [CrossRef]
19. Shen, J.; Moats, R.A.; Pollack, H.A.; Robinson, M.R.; Attar, M. Distribution of 14C-Latanoprost Following a Single Intracameral Administration Versus Repeated Topical Administration. *Ophthalmol. Ther.* **2020**, *9*, 929–940. [CrossRef]
20. Pérez-Roca, F.; Rodrigo-Morales, E.; Garzón, I.; Oliveira, A.C.; Martín-Piedra, M.; Carriel, V.; Ortiz-Pérez, A.I.; Sánchez-Montesinos, I.; Campos, A.; Alaminos, M. Effects of Four Formulations of Prostaglandin Analogs on Eye Surface Cells. A Comparative Study. *PLoS ONE* **2015**, *10*, e0129419. [CrossRef]
21. Esaki, Y.; Shimazaki, A.; Pellinen, P. Ocular Tolerability of Preservative-Free Tafluprost and Latanoprost: In vitro and in vivo Comparative Study. *Open Ophthalmol. J.* **2016**, *10*, 146–153. [CrossRef]
22. Ayyala, R.S.; Zurakowski, D.; Smith, J.A.; Monshizadeh, R.; Netland, P.A.; Richards, D.W.; Layden, W.E. A clinical study of the Ahmed glaucoma valve implant in advanced glaucoma. *Ophthalmology* **1998**, *105*, 1968–1976. [CrossRef] [PubMed]
23. Nouri-Mahdavi, K.; Caprioli, J. Evaluation of the hypertensive phase after insertion of the Ahmed Glaucoma Valve. *Am. J. Ophthalmol.* **2003**, *136*, 1001–1008. [CrossRef] [PubMed]
24. Jeong, H.J.; Park, H.Y.L.; Park, C.K. Effects of Early Postoperative Intraocular Pressure after Ahmed Glaucoma Valve Implantation on Long-term Surgical Outcomes. *Korean J. Ophthalmol.* **2018**, *32*, 391–399. [CrossRef] [PubMed]

Journal of
Clinical Medicine

MDPI

Article

Effect of Visual Field Test on Intraocular Pressure in Glaucoma Patients

Weon Jin Jang [1], Han Jun Chung [2], Min Woo Lee [2], Jung Tae Kim [2], Hyung-Bin Lim [3] and Kee Sup Park [4,5,*]

1 Department of Public Health, Graduate School of Konyang University, Daejeon 35365, Republic of Korea; jwj7677@naver.com
2 Department of Ophthalmology, Konyang University College of Medicine, Daejeon 35365, Republic of Korea; hanjuncyayo@gmail.com (H.J.C.); bogus1105@gmail.com (M.W.L.); 200679@kyuh.ac.kr (J.T.K.)
3 1.0 Eye Clinic, Daejeon 34946, Republic of Korea; cromfans@hanmail.net
4 Department of Ophthalmology, Chungnam National University College of Medicine, Daejeon 35015, Republic of Korea
5 Myunggok Medical Research Institute, Konyang University, Daejeon 35365, Republic of Korea
* Correspondence: red-mirr@hanmail.net; Tel.: +82-42-280-8433; Fax: +82-42-255-3745

Abstract: Objectives: To evaluate changes in intraocular pressure (IOP) before versus after a visual field test in glaucoma patients. **Methods:** A total of 132 patients with glaucoma and 103 control subjects who visited Konyang University Hospital between August 2024 and May 2025 were included in the study. the right eye of each patient was selected for analysis. Visual field tests were conducted using the Humphrey Visual Field (HVF) analyzer (Zeiss Humphrey, San Leandro, CA, USA) with the SITA standard program (Central 24-2). Intraocular pressure was measured by two ophthalmologists at five time points: before the test and immediately, 10 min, 30 min, and 60 min after the test. **Results:** The average intraocular pressure decreased from 15.09 mmHg before the test to 14.29 mmHg immediately afterward; it declined further to 13.59 mmHg at 10 min in glaucoma patients. It then gradually increased to 15.01 mmHg at 60 min, returning to pre-test levels. Participants were divided into three age groups (40s, 50s, and 60s) for analysis. Across all groups, the IOP followed a similar pattern: a significant decrease for up to 10 min, followed by recovery at 60 min. Although a reduction in IOP was also observed in the control group after visual field testing, the magnitude of the decrease was smaller compared to the glaucoma patients. **Conclusions:** IOP declined immediately after the visual field test and remained lower for up to 10 min. It subsequently returned to baseline by 60 min. Therefore, when measuring the IOP after a visual field test, there is no need to adjust for temporary fluctuations if the measurement is performed 60 min after the test.

Keywords: glaucoma; intraocular pressure; visual field test

1. Introduction

Glaucoma comprises a group of progressive optic neuropathies characterized by structural damage to the optic nerve accompanied by corresponding visual field loss. Elevated intraocular pressure (IOP) is the most significant risk factor, and lowering IOP remains the primary therapeutic strategy [1].

IOP is regulated by the continuous flow of aqueous humor and plays a key role in maintaining the eye's structural integrity and visual function. Normal IOP ranges from 10 to 21 mmHg, with an average of 15 mmHg [2]. Elevated IOP is the strongest risk factor for glaucoma; lowering the IOP is the only proven treatment for slowing or preventing optic nerve damage [3]. Various factors influence IOP, including age, sex, ethnicity, diurnal fluctuations, systemic hemodynamics, exercise, positional changes, refractive errors, and medications [4–7]. Although a high IOP contributes to glaucoma by damaging the optic nerve, the precise mechanisms underlying IOP elevation remain unclear [8–11].

The visual field test is a crucial diagnostic tool for assessing glaucoma progression by measuring the extent of visual field defects. It is particularly important in early-stage glaucoma when the visual field may only be partially affected [12,13].

However, there is ongoing debate regarding the relationship between the visual field test and IOP. Previous studies have yielded conflicting results. Bertaud et al. [14] and Adhikari et al. [15] found no significant difference in IOP values before and after the exam, suggesting the minimal physiological influence of the test. In contrast, Lee et al. [16] reported a temporary increase 10 min after the exam, which normalized within 20 min. Similarly, Sawada et al. [17] observed a significant decrease in IOP after the exam. Other studies have reported transient elevations; for instance, Ni et al. [18] found that the IOP increased after testing 22.9% of glaucoma patients, with a more than 20% change in some cases. Li et al. [19] and Recupero et al. [20] also described short-term IOP elevations that returned to baseline within an hour. Moreover, Asrani et al. [21] emphasized that the IOP can fluctuate widely in glaucoma patients, even when the mean values remain within the normal range. Liu et al. [22] further demonstrated that IOP fluctuations were more pronounced in glaucomatous eyes than in healthy eyes, highlighting the importance of understanding dynamic IOP behavior during visual field testing.

Given the lack of conclusive evidence regarding IOP fluctuations and influencing factors, we investigated fluctuations in the IOP in relation to the test and identified specific factors that may drive these changes.

2. Methods

2.1. Patients

We examined the right eyes of 132 outpatients with open-angle glaucoma and 103 in a control group who visited Konyang University Hospital between August 2024 and May 2025. All glaucoma patients had an open angle confirmed by gonioscopy, glaucomatous optic nerve damage with corresponding visual field defects, and maintained normal IOP while using anti-glaucoma eye drops. The control group consisted of normal patients who visited a glaucoma clinic. Visual field tests meeting reliability criteria (gaze loss $\leq$ 20%, false-negative responses $\leq$ 15%, and false-positive responses $\leq$ 15%) were included in the analysis. Patients with corneal disease, post-cataract surgery status, or post-glaucoma surgery status were excluded. This prospective study was approved by the Institutional Review Board of Konyang University Hospital in the Republic of Korea (IRB number: 2024-05-023-001). It was conducted in accordance with all relevant requirements of the Declaration of Helsinki. Informed consent was acquired from all participants.

2.2. Humphrey Visual Field (HVF)

Humphrey Visual Field (HVF) testing (Zeiss Humphrey, San Leandro, CA, USA—SITA standard program, Central 24-2) was used as a quantitative visual field assessment. Patients with dilated pupils were excluded, and myopia was corrected prior to testing.

2.3. Intraocular Pressure (IOP)

IOP measurements were obtained from patients attending the glaucoma clinic by two experienced ophthalmologists using the Goldmann applanation tonometer (GAT) (model

AT 900, Haag-Streit International, Köniz, Switzerland) at five time points: before the visual field test and immediately, 10 min, 30 min, and 60 min after the test. All measurements were performed under standardized conditions using consistent techniques. Both examiners were glaucoma specialists trained in GAT measurement protocols, and the same equipment was used throughout the study. For staining, 0.5% paracaine (Hanmi Medicine, Seoul, Republic of Korea) and fluorescein strips were applied. For each examination, the average of two consecutive IOP measurements was used for statistical analysis. To assess inter-observer reliability, the intraclass correlation coefficient (ICC) was calculated for baseline IOP measurements. The results demonstrated excellent agreement between the two examiners, with an ICC of 0.982 in the glaucoma group and 0.977 in the control group, indicating high consistency and reliability in the measurement process.

2.4. Optical Coherence Tomography (OCT)

An experienced examiner performed OCT measurements using a Cirrus HD OCT 6000 (Carl Zeiss Meditec, Dublin, CA, USA; version 10.0). The 200 × 200 optic disk cube scanning protocol was applied to assess RNFL thickness. We focused on RNFL thickness rather than the ganglion cell layer (GCL) because RNFL is a widely accepted and reproducible marker for detecting early glaucomatous damage. It shows strong correlation with disease progression and is less affected by macular pathology compared to GCL analysis. Moreover, RNFL thinning often appears earlier than ganglion cell loss in the disease course [23].

2.5. Statistical Analysis

Statistical analyses were conducted using PASW software, version 27.0 (SPSS Inc., Chicago, IL, USA); demographic characteristics were compared between the two groups using Student's t-test and chi-square test. Changes in IOP were analyzed with repeated-measures analysis of variance along with univariate and multivariate linear mixed models. A p-value < 0.05 was considered statistically significant. In the univariate model, age, sex, and a history of diabetes mellitus and hypertension were assessed to determine their influence on changes in IOP. The multivariate model examined variables identified in univariate analysis, while also incorporating additional independent factors to assess their unique effects.

3. Results

3.1. Demographics

The study included a total of 132 eyes from glaucoma patients and 103 from a control group. The mean age was 58.66 ± 1.36 years for glaucoma patients and 59.26 ± 1.85 years for the control group ($p = 0.620$). There were no significant differences between the two groups in hypertension, DM, sex, axial length, baseline IOP, CCT, BCVA, spherical equivalent, and axial length (all Ps > 0.05; Table 1). Glaucoma patients used an average of 1.52 ± 0.11 anti-glaucoma eye drops. The mean RNFL thickness was thinner in the glaucoma patients than in the control group (80.58 ± 1.41 μm vs. 97.80 ± 7.61 μm, $p < 0.001$).

HVF testing was performed, and the average testing time was significantly longer in glaucoma patients than in the control group (5.71 ± 0.13 min vs. 4.81 ± 0.15 min, $p < 0.001$). The MD measures overall visual field sensitivity loss and is categorized into three stages: early (−2 to −6 dB), moderate (−6 to −12 dB), and advanced (<−12 dB) [24]. Our glaucoma patients had an average MD of −3.02 ± 0.59 dB, consistent with early-stage glaucoma. The pattern for standard deviation was significantly higher in the glaucoma patients compared with the control group (4.56 ± 0.42 dB, 1.98 ± 0.93 dB, and $p < 0.001$). The VFI was lower in glaucoma patients than in the control group (91.88 ± 1.63%. vs. 97.69 ± 2.02%, $p < 0.001$).

Table 1. Demographic characteristics of patients.

	Glaucoma Patients	Control Group	p-Value *
Number of patients	132	103	
Age (year, mean ±SD)	58.66 ± 1.36	59.26 ± 1.85	0.432
Sex (male, %)	64 (48.4)	53 (51.5)	0.537 †
Hypertension (%)	19 (14.3)	16 (15.5)	0.795 †
DM (%)	12 (9.1)	11 (10.7)	0.852 †
IOP-lowering medication (n)	1.52 ± 0.11	0	0.001
Baseline IOP	15.09 ± 2.24	15.04 ± 2.14	0.844
CCT (mean ± SD)	521.79 ± 5.93	519 ± 4.38	0.580
BCVA (logMAR, mean ± SD)	0.027 ± 0.01	0.023 ± 0.01	0.549
Spherical equivalent (diopter, mean ± SD)	−1.14 ± 0.32	−1.09 ± 0.34	0.534
Axial length (mm, mean ± SD)	23.15 ± 0.11	23.30 ± 0.21	0.155
Mean RNFL thickness (µm, mean ± SD)	80.58 ± 1.41	97.80 ± 7.61	0.001
Humphrey visual field			
Mean deviation (dB)	−3.02 ± 0.59	−0.93 ± 0.36	0.001
Pattern standard deviation (dB)	4.56 ± 0.42	1.98 ± 0.93	0.001
Visual field index (%)	91.88 ± 1.63	97.69 ± 2.02	0.001
VF testing time (min, mean ± SD)	5.71 ± 0.13	4.81 ± 0.15	0.001

* p-value from Student's t-test, † p-value from the chi-squared test.

3.2. Relationship Between IOP Before Versus After the Visual Field Test

Table 2 and Figure 1 show changes in the IOP according to time point after the exam. The mean IOP was 15.09 ± 2.24 mmHg. Although IOP in the glaucoma patients and control group significantly decreased immediately after the exam, as well as at 10 min and 30 min, it returned to baseline by 60 min. As shown in Figure 1, the difference in IOP before and after the test were statistically significant ($p < 0.001$); the lowest pressure was observed 10 min after the exam. Changes in IOP over time were statistically significant ($p < 0.001$) for both glaucoma patients and the control group. Overall, changes in IOP over time were statistically significant ($p < 0.001$) in both groups. The maximum IOP difference in glaucoma patients and the control group was −1.5 mmHg and −0.53 mmHg, respectively, indicating that the change in IOP was greater in glaucoma patients.

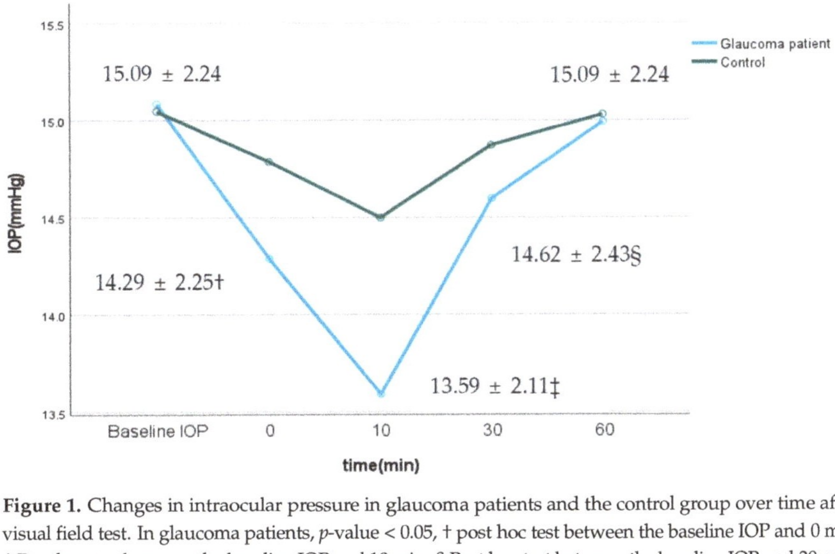

Figure 1. Changes in intraocular pressure in glaucoma patients and the control group over time after visual field test. In glaucoma patients, p-value < 0.05, † post hoc test between the baseline IOP and 0 min. ‡ Post hoc test between the baseline IOP and 10 min. § Post hoc test between the baseline IOP and 30 min.

Table 2. Comparison of IOP variations between before (baseline) and after (0, 10, 30, and 60 min) visual field testing.

	Baseline IOP	0 min	10 min	30 min	60 min	p-Value *
Glaucoma patients (n = 132)	15.09 ± 2.24	14.29 ± 2.25	13.59 ± 2.11	14.62 ± 2.43	15.01 ± 2.18	**<0.001**
Control group (n = 103)	15.04 ± 2.14	14.79 ± 2.06	14.51 ± 2.01	14.85 ± 2.34	15.02 ± 2.19	**<0.001**
						<0.001

* p-value from the repeated-measures ANOVA (analysis of variation). Significant p-values are bolded.

3.3. Relationship Between IOP Before Versus After the Visual Field Test, According to Age

A total of 18 eyes from patients in their 40s, 20 eyes from those in their 50s, and 28 eyes from those in their 60s were analyzed. Table 3 and Figure 2 show age-related fluctuations in IOP over time.

Table 3. Comparison of IOP variation between before (baseline) and after (0, 10, 30, and 60 min) visual field testing by ages.

Time		Baseline IOP	0 min	10 min	30 min	60 min	p-Value *
	40 s (n = 38)	14.83 ± 2.28	14.16 ± 2.19	13.33 ± 2.24	14.50 ± 2.29	14.78 ± 2.28	**<0.001**
Age groups	50 s (n = 40)	15.15 ± 1.81	14.15 ± 1.95	13.50 ± 1.88	14.45 ± 1.90	15.05 ± 1.85	**<0.001**
	60 s (n = 54)	15.21 ± 2.54	14.46 ± 2.49	13.82 ± 2.17	14.82 ± 2.54	15.11 ± 2.36	**<0.001**

* p-value from the repeated-measures ANOVA (analysis of variation). Significant p-values are bolded.

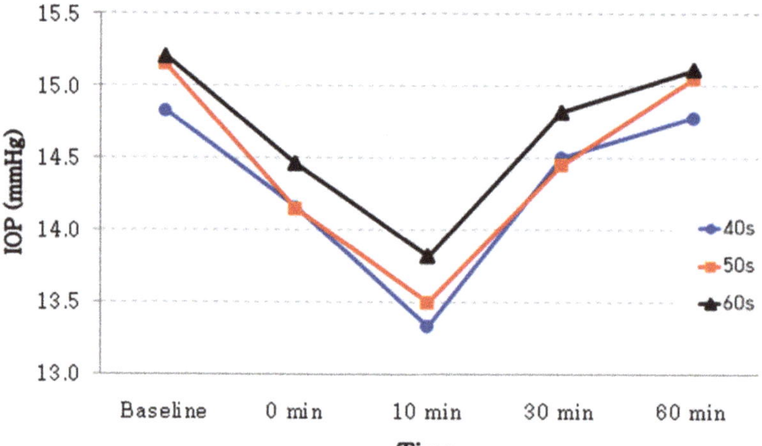

Figure 2. Changes in intraocular pressure over time after visual field test by age group.

In summary, the average IOP of patients in their 60s (15.21 ± 2.54 mmHg) was significantly higher than that of those in their 40s (14.83 ± 2.28 mmHg). Additionally, the decrease in IOP 10 min after the exam was greater among patients in their 40s (−8.98%) than among those in their 60s (−9.08%). Finally, in every age group, the post-exam IOP was significantly lower than the pre-exam value (p < 0.001; Table 3).

3.4. Factors Influencing Changes in IOP

According to univariate and multivariate linear mixed models, the patient's age, sex, diabetes, hypertension, use of glaucoma eye drops, average corneal thickness, axial length, spherical equivalent, VFI, MD, and average retinal nerve fiber layer (RNFL) thickness significantly affected changes in IOP (Table 4). In the univariate model, age, hypertension, and average RNFL thickness were significant factors at $p \leq 0.1$. In the multivariate model, female patients, those with hypertension, and those with thicker RNFLs had lower average IOPs (Table 4).

Table 4. Univariate and multivariate linear mixed-effect model determination of factors associated with changes in the IOP.

	Univariate		Multivariate	
Factors	**Estimate (95% CI)**	***p*-Value**	**Estimate (95% CI)**	***p*-Value**
Age	−0.003 (−0.05 to 0.06)	0.119		
Sex (1 = male, 2 = female)	−1.375 (−2.47 to −0.29)	**0.014**	−1.415 (−2.45 to −0.38)	**0.008**
DM	0.114 (−1.63 to 1.86)	0.897		
HTN	−1.079 (−2.26 to 0.10)	**0.073**	−1.231 (−2.34 to −0.12)	**0.030**
IOP-lowering medication	0.281 (−0.37 to 0.93)	0.390		
Central cornea thickness	−0.005 (−0.02 to 0.01)	0.415		
Axial length	−0.333 (−1.07 to 0.40)	0.368		
BCVA(LogMAR)	−4.504 (−12.75 to 3.74)	0.279		
Spherical equivalent	0.069 (−0.16 to 0.29)	0.599		
Visual field index	0.012 (−0.03 to 0.06)	0.583		
Mean deviation	0.071 (−0.05 to 0.19)	0.259		
Pattern standard deviation	−0.107 (−0.28 to 0.07)	0.229		
Average RNFL	−0.046 (−0.09 to 0.003)	**0.069**	−0.057 (−0.10 to −0.01)	**0.017**

IOP = intraocular pressure, BCVA = best corrected visual acuity, logMAR = logarithm of the minimum angle of resolution, RNFL = retinal nerve fiber layer, and Significant *p*-values are bolded ($p < 0.1$).

4. Discussion

In glaucoma, elevated IOP can impair ocular blood circulation and cause optic nerve damage, potentially resulting in complete blindness. The global prevalence of glaucoma continues to rise. Previous studies have shown that patients with glaucoma have an impaired autoregulation of ocular blood flow in response to changes in blood pressure or IOP compared with healthy individuals [25,26]. The measurement of IOP and visual field testing is essential for monitoring disease progression and guiding treatment decisions. Visual field testing is typically performed before the clinical consultation to allow for comparison with previous results.

IOP changes following visual field testing warrant careful consideration. In this study, we measured the IOP at multiple time points (0, 10, 30, and 60 min after the test) and found that it decreased after testing but returned to baseline by 60 min. Table 2 and Figure 1 present the changes in IOP in both glaucoma patients and controls. Both groups demonstrated a transient reduction in the IOP immediately after visual field testing, with statistically significant differences ($p < 0.001$). In the glaucoma group, the maximum reduction occurred at 10 min post-test, with a mean decrease of approximately −1.5 mmHg, followed by a gradual return to near-baseline levels by 60 min. In contrast, the control group exhibited a smaller maximum decrease of about −0.5 mmHg. The more pronounced IOP fluctuation observed in glaucoma patients may reflect impaired ocular blood flow autoregulation. Previous studies have reported that patients with glaucoma show compromised autoregulatory responses to changes in ocular perfusion pressure or IOP [25–27]. This reduced capacity for autoregulation may render them more susceptible to physiological stress induced by visual field testing. Although statistically significant IOP changes were also observed in the control group, the absolute magnitude was minimal and recovered rapidly. This suggests that homeostatic mechanisms involving the autonomic nervous system and trabecular meshwork function are better preserved in healthy eyes, resulting in superior IOP recovery compared with glaucoma patients. These findings are relevant not only for the diagnosis and monitoring of glaucoma, but also for patient counseling. Patients can be reassured that post-test IOP fluctuations are transient, decrease within a short period, and eventually return to baseline.

Our findings differ from previous studies that reported increases in IOP after the test. For example, Li et al. [19] found that the IOPs of 31 open-angle glaucoma patients (62 eyes) significantly increased by 12.7% immediately after the test. Similar findings were reported by Recupero et al. [20], who studied 49 primary open-angle glaucoma patients (94 eyes). The mean IOP change was 2.38 ± 3.49 mmHg. However, in both studies, the IOP returned to baseline within 1 h after the exam, as observed in our study. Additionally, Recupero et al. [20] reported higher IOPs in younger patients, which is consistent with our findings.

Our findings are consistent with those of Sawada et al. [17], who also observed a decrease in the IOP after visual field testing in patients with open-angle glaucoma. In their study, the IOP of the right eye decreased from 12.8 ± 2.9 mmHg to 12.3 ± 2.6 mmHg, whereas the left eye remained relatively stable (12.6 ± 2.8 mmHg to 12.5 ± 2.6 mmHg). This difference may be attributable to the right eye being tested first. The reduction in IOP may result from near focusing, which induces ciliary muscle contraction and subsequently enhances aqueous humor outflow [7,24,28]. Similarly, Cassidy et al. [29] reported that in glaucoma patients, engaging in near work for 10 min produced a significant decrease in the IOP compared with looking at a distance for the same duration, a finding in agreement with our results.

As shown in Table 3 and Figure 2, we also found that the IOP was higher in older patients: 14.83 ± 2.28 mmHg among patients in their 40s versus 15.21 ± 2.54 mmHg among those in their 60s. Caprioli et al. [30] reported a relationship between older age and various physiological and structural changes that can increase the IOP. They found that trabecular meshwork dysfunction, changes in lens size, biodynamic alterations in the posterior eye, decreases in retinal ganglion cells, and reduced intracranial pressure were major factors contributing to an elevated IOP. This increase may be due to reduced aqueous humor drainage caused by accommodation dysfunction [20,24]. Psychological stress and nervousness during the test may also contribute due to its demanding nature [31]. The IOP could decrease when the patient relaxes after the exam. Lee et al. [16] reported a significant decrease in IOP 10 min after the exam, followed by a quick recovery within 20 min. This may be attributed to the lower average age of their patients (57.4 ± 11.3 years) relative to ours (58.66 ± 1.36 years).

In this study, we used a univariate model to discover that sex, hypertension, and average RNFL thickness (p-value < 0.1)) affect IOP and then used a multivariate model for additional analysis. We found that age, hypertension, and average RNFL thickness were significantly associated with IOP changes (p-value < 0.05). Several previous studies have suggested that postmenopausal hormonal therapy in women may contribute to reduced IOP levels [32–34]. While our study did not collect specific data regarding hormonal status or therapy, the age distribution of our female participants (predominantly in their 40s to 60s) overlaps with the age group commonly undergoing menopausal transition. Thus, hormonal influences may be one of several factors contributing to IOP differences in this population, though further investigation is required. We also observed that the average IOP of hypertensive patients (14.82 ± 2.04 mmHg) was lower than that of non-hypertensive patients (15.23 ± 2.35 mmHg). This difference may be related to the effects of systemic anti-hypertensive medications, which have been reported to lower ocular perfusion pressure and IOP in some prior studies [26]. However, as detailed information on medication use and blood pressure control was not collected, the interpretation of these findings should be approached with caution. The assessment of RNFL thickness is valuable in evaluating glaucoma progression. A thicker RNFL generally reflects a healthier retina, whereas thinning is an early marker of disease progression [35–37]. In our study, patients with a greater average RNFL thickness exhibited less fluctuation in IOP [38].

This study focused on patients with early-stage glaucoma. According to the Early Manifest Glaucoma Trial (EMGT) [39], the risk of glaucoma progression can be reduced by approximately 10% with each 1 mmHg decrease in IOP. In our study, no increase in IOP was observed following visual field testing. These findings may help reassure patients by alleviating concerns about IOP fluctuations after visual field examinations.

This study has several limitations. First, it included only patients with early-stage, open-angle glaucoma; therefore, the findings may not be generalizable to individuals with advanced glaucoma, angle-closure glaucoma, or secondary glaucoma. Second, although we assessed IOP fluctuations after visual field testing, we did not investigate concurrent biometric changes in anterior segment structures, such as anterior chamber depth, lens thickness, or lens position. Third, the follow-up duration was limited to 60 min, which may have missed delayed IOP responses. Fourth, we did not include measurements of the ganglion cell layer (GCL) or assess correlations with other imaging modalities such as optical coherence tomography angiography (OCT-A), which may have provided additional structural insights. Lastly, potential influences such as psychological stress or fatigue during the test—which could affect IOP—were not evaluated.

Despite these limitations, this study has several strengths. Repeated IOP measurements at multiple time points allowed for a robust assessment of temporal changes following visual field testing. Moreover, the inclusion of a control group enabled direct comparisons, highlighting the distinct IOP responses observed in glaucoma patients.

In conclusion, our study indicated that the IOP did not increase before or after visual field testing, eliminating concerns about such effects. Although there was a significant decrease 10 min after the exam, the IOP returned to baseline by 60 min. Therefore, measuring a patient's IOP 60 min after a visual field test allows for a more accurate assessment. However, patients with mid- to late-stage glaucoma will require further follow-up.

Author Contributions: Design and conduct of the study (K.S.P., W.J.J. and J.T.K.); Collection of data (W.J.J., H.-B.L. and M.W.L.); Analysis and interpretation of data (K.S.P., W.J.J., H.J.C., M.W.L., H.-B.L. and J.T.K.); Writing the article (K.S.P. and W.J.J.); Critical revision of the article (K.S.P., W.J.J. and M.W.L.); Final approval of the article (K.S.P., W.J.J., H.-B.L. and M.W.L.). All authors have read and agreed to the published version of the manuscript.

Funding: This work was supported by Konyang University Myunggok Research Fund of 2024-01.

Institutional Review Board Statement: The study was conducted according to the guidelines of the Declaration of Helsinki, and approved by the Institutional Review Board of Konyang University Hospital in Daejeon, Republic of Korea (IRB number: 2024-05-023-001: approval date: 14 August 2024).

Informed Consent Statement: Informed consent was obtained from all subjects involved in the study.

Data Availability Statement: The original contributions presented in this study are included in the article. Further inquiries can be directed to the corresponding author.

Conflicts of Interest: The authors declare no conflicts of interest.

References

1. Agarwal, R.; Gupta, S.K.; Agarwal, P.; Saxena, R.; Agrawal, S.S. Current concepts in the pathophysiology of glaucoma. *Indian J. Ophthalmol.* **2009**, *57*, 257–266. [CrossRef] [PubMed]
2. Gabelt, B.; Kaufman, P. Aqueous humor hydrodynamics. In *Adler's Physiology of the Eye: Clinical Application*; Mosby: St. Louis, MO, USA, 2003.
3. Allingham, R.R.; Damji, K.F.; Freedman, S.F.; Moroi, S.E.; Rhee, D.J.; Shields, M.B. *Shields Textbook of Glaucoma*; Lippincott Williams & Wilkins: Philadelphia, PA, USA, 2012.
4. Ha, A.; Kim, Y.K.; Park, Y.J.; Jeoung, J.W.; Park, K.H. Intraocular pressure change during reading or writing on smartphone. *PLoS ONE* **2018**, *13*, e0206061. [CrossRef]
5. Ahn, J.H.; Kil, H.K.; Lee, M.V. Positional Change of Intraocular Pressure and Its Relationship to Ocular Pulse Amplitude. *J. Korean Ophthalmol. Soc.* **2015**, *56*, 234–240. [CrossRef]
6. Pakravan, M.; Samaeili, A.; Esfandiari, H.; Hassanpour, K.; Hooshmandi, S.; Yazdani, S.; Sharifipour, F.; Doozandeh, A.; Einollahi, B.; Pakravan, P.; et al. The influence of near vision tasks on intraocular pressure in normal subjects and glaucoma patients. *J. Ophthalmic Vis. Res.* **2022**, *17*, 497. [CrossRef] [PubMed]
7. Priluck, A.Z.; Hoie, A.B.; High, R.R.; Gulati, V.; Ghate, D.A. Effect of near work on intraocular pressure in emmetropes. *J. Ophthalmol.* **2020**, *2020*, 1352434. [CrossRef]
8. He, M.; Foster, P.J.; Ge, J.; Huang, W.; Zheng, Y.; Friedman, D.S.; Lee, P.S.; Khaw, P.T. Prevalence and clinical characteristics of glaucoma in adult Chinese: A population-based study in Liwan District, Guangzhou. *Investig. Ophthalmol. Vis. Sci.* **2006**, *47*, 2782–2788. [CrossRef]
9. Khaw, P.; Elkington, A. Glaucoma—1: Diagnosis. *BMJ* **2004**, *328*, 97–99. [CrossRef]
10. Orzalesi, N.; Rossetti, L.; Bottoli, A.; Fogagnolo, P. Comparison of the effects of latanoprost, travoprost, and bimatoprost on circadian intraocular pressure in patients with glaucoma or ocular hypertension. *Ophthalmology* **2006**, *113*, 239–246. [CrossRef]
11. Danesh-Meyer, H.V.; Boland, M.V.; Savino, P.J.; Miller, N.R.; Subramanian, P.S.; Girkin, C.A.; Quigley, H.A. Optic disc morphology in open-angle glaucoma compared with anterior ischemic optic neuropathies. *Investig. Ophthalmol. Vis. Sci.* **2010**, *51*, 2003–2010. [CrossRef]
12. Stewart, W.C.; Shields, M.B. The peripheral visual field in glaucoma: Reevaluation in the age of automated perimetry. *Surv. Ophthalmol.* **1991**, *36*, 59–69. [CrossRef]
13. Odden, J.L.; Mihailovic, A.; Boland, M.V.; Friedman, D.S.; West, S.K.; Ramulu, P.Y. Evaluation of central and peripheral visual field concordance in glaucoma. *Investig. Ophthalmol. Vis. Sci.* **2016**, *57*, 2797–2804. [CrossRef] [PubMed]
14. Bertaud, S.; Skarbek Borowski, E.; Abbas, R.; Baudouin, C.; Labbé, A. Influence of automated visual field testing on intraocular pressure. *BMC Ophthalmol.* **2020**, *20*, 363. [CrossRef]
15. Adhikari, P.G.; Joshi, S.N.; Poudel, A. Influence of visual field testing on intraocular pressure in patients with glaucoma suspects attending tertiary care center in Kathmandu. *J. Chitwan Med. Coll.* **2023**, *13*, 53–56. [CrossRef]
16. Lee, C.M.; Yoo, Y.C. Short-Term Effect of Standard Automated Perimetry Testing on Intraocular Pressure in Patients with Open-Angle Glaucoma. *Int. Sch. Res. Not.* **2013**, *2013*, 956504. [CrossRef]
17. Sawada, A.; Yamada, H.; Yamamoto, Y.; Yamamoto, T. Intraocular pressure alterations after visual field testing. *Jpn. J. Ophthalmol.* **2014**, *58*, 429–434. [CrossRef]
18. Ni, N.; Tsai, J.C.; Shields, M.B.; Loewen, N.A. Elevation of intraocular pressure in glaucoma patients after automated visual field testing. *J. Glaucoma* **2012**, *21*, 590–595. [CrossRef] [PubMed]
19. Li, M.; Zheng, B.; Wang, Q.; Sun, X. Impact of visual field testing on intraocular pressure change trends in healthy people and glaucoma patients. *J. Ophthalmol.* **2020**, *2020*, 7936205. [CrossRef] [PubMed]
20. Recupero, S.M.; Contestabile, M.T.; Taverniti, L.; Villani, G.M.; Recupero, V. Open-angle glaucoma: Variations in the intraocular pressure after visual field examination. *J. Glaucoma* **2003**, *12*, 114–118. [CrossRef]
21. Asrani, S.G.; McGlumphy, E.J.; Al-Aswad, L.A.; Chaya, C.J.; Lin, S.; Musch, D.C.; Pitha, I.; Robin, A.L.; Wirostko, B.; Johnson, T.V. The relationship between intraocular pressure and glaucoma: An evolving concept. *Prog. Retin. Eye Res.* **2024**, *103*, 101303. [CrossRef]
22. Liu, T.; Cai, Y.; Hu, M.; Wang, Z.; Liu, X.; Chen, M.; Wang, K. The impact of intraocular pressure fluctuations on the progression of glaucoma and associated factors. *Adv. Ophthalmol. Pract. Res.* **2025**, *5*, 142–148. [CrossRef] [PubMed]
23. Soliman, T.T.; Abd Abd Gad, E.; Selim, S.M. Ganglion cell analysis versus retinal nerve fiber layer thickness in glaucoma diagnosis. *J. Egypt. Ophthalmol. Soc.* **2019**, *112*, 122–129. [CrossRef]
24. Armaly, M.F.; Rubin, M.L. Accommodation and applanation tonometry. *Arch. Ophthalmol.* **1961**, *65*, 415–423. [CrossRef]
25. Gherghel, D.; Orgül, S.; Gugleta, K.; Gekkieva, M.; Flammer, J. Relationship between ocular perfusion pressure and retrobulbar blood flow in patients with glaucoma with progressive damage. *Am. J. Ophthalmol.* **2000**, *130*, 597–605. [CrossRef]

26. Flammer, J.; Orgül, S.; Costa, V.P.; Orzalesi, N.; Krieglstein, G.K.; Serra, L.M.; Renard, J.-P.; Stefánsson, E. The impact of ocular blood flow in glaucoma. *Prog. Retin. Eye Res.* **2002**, *21*, 359–393. [CrossRef] [PubMed]
27. Schmidl, D.; Garhofer, G.; Schmetterer, L. The complex interaction between ocular perfusion pressure and ocular blood flow–relevance for glaucoma. *Exp. Eye Res.* **2011**, *93*, 141–155. [CrossRef]
28. Mauger, R.R.; Likens, C.P.; Applebaum, M. Effects of accommodation and repeated applanation tonometry on intraocular pressure. *Optom. Vis. Sci.* **1984**, *61*, 28–30. [CrossRef] [PubMed]
29. Cassidy, L.; Delaney, Y.; Fitzpatrick, P.; Blake, J. Effect of accommodation on intraocular pressure in glaucomatous eyes. *Ir. J. Med. Sci.* **1998**, *167*, 17–18. [CrossRef]
30. Caprioli, J. Glaucoma: A disease of early cellular senescence. *Investig. Ophthalmol. Vis. Sci.* **2013**, *54*, ORSF60–ORSF67. [CrossRef]
31. Erb, C.; Brody, S.; Rau, H. Effect of mental and physical stress on intraocular pressure—A pilot study. *Klin. Monatsblatter Fur Augenheilkd.* **1998**, *212*, 270–274. [CrossRef]
32. Sator, M.O.; Joura, E.A.; Frigo, P.; Kurz, C.; Metka, M.; Hommer, A.; Huber, J.C. Hormone replacement therapy and intraocular pressure. *Maturitas* **1997**, *28*, 55–58. [CrossRef]
33. Sator, M.O.; Akramian, J.; Joura, E.A.; Nessmann, A.; Wedrich, A.; Gruber, D.; Metka, M.; Huber, J.C. Reduction of intraocular pressure in a glaucoma patient undergoing hormone replacement therapy. *Maturitas* **1998**, *29*, 93–95. [CrossRef]
34. Affinito, P.; Sardo, A.D.S.; Di Carlo, C.; Sammartino, A.; Tommaselli, G.A.; Bifulco, G.; Loffredo, A.; Loffredo, M.; Nappi, C. Effects of hormone replacement therapy on ocular function in postmenopause. *Menopause* **2003**, *10*, 482–487. [CrossRef] [PubMed]
35. Quigley, H.A.; Katz, J.; Derick, R.J.; Gilbert, D.; Sommer, A. An evaluation of optic disc and nerve fiber layer examinations in monitoring progression of early glaucoma damage. *Ophthalmology* **1992**, *99*, 19–28. [CrossRef] [PubMed]
36. Sommer, A.; Quigley, H.A.; Robin, A.L.; Miller, N.R.; Katz, J.; Arkell, S. Evaluation of nerve fiber layer assessment. *Arch. Ophthalmol.* **1984**, *102*, 1766–1771. [CrossRef] [PubMed]
37. Quigly, H. Optic nerve damage in human glaucoma, III Quantitative correlative correlation of nerve fiber loss and visual field defects in glaucoma, ischemic neuropathy, papilledema and toxic neuropathy. *Arch. Ophthalmol.* **1982**, *100*, 135–146. [CrossRef]
38. Nishida, T.; Moghimi, S.; Chang, A.C.; Walker, E.; Liebmann, J.M.; Fazio, M.A.; Girkin, C.A.; Zangwill, L.M.; Weinreb, R.N. Association of intraocular pressure with retinal nerve fiber layer thinning in patients with glaucoma. *JAMA Ophthalmol.* **2022**, *140*, 1209–1216. [CrossRef]
39. Leske, M.C.; Heijl, A.; Hyman, L.; Bengtsson, B.; Group, E.M.G.T. Early Manifest Glaucoma Trial: Design and baseline data. *Ophthalmology* **1999**, *106*, 2144–2153. [CrossRef]

Journal of
Clinical Medicine

MDPI

Article

Intraluminal 10-0 Nylon Stenting in PRESERFLO™ MicroShunt Surgery for Pseudoexfoliation Glaucoma

Miranda Gehrke, Leonie F. Keidel, Lara Buhl, Siegfried G. Priglinger and Marc J. Mackert *

Department of Ophthalmology, LMU University Hospital, LMU Munich, Mathildenstr. 8, 80336 Munich, Germany; miranda.gehrke@med.uni-muenchen.de (M.G.); leonie.keidel@med.uni-muenchen.de (L.F.K.); lara.buhl@med.uni-muenchen.de (L.B.); siegfried.priglinger@med.uni-muenchen.de (S.G.P.)

* Correspondence: marc.mackert@med.uni-muenchen.de

Abstract: Background/Objectives: Early postoperative hypotony and complications like choroidal detachment can occur after Preserflo MicroShunt (MS) implantation in patients with pseudoexfoliation glaucoma (PEXG). To prevent these risks, outflow from the microshunt tube can be reduced by implementing a nylon stent. This study aims to evaluate the impact of intraluminal stenting of the MS during the first four months after surgery. **Methods:** This retrospective study of 43 eyes investigated the incidence of intraocular hypotony in PEXG patients undergoing MS implantation with (n = 23) or without (n = 20) intraluminal stenting using a 10.0 nylon suture. The follow-up period was four months after surgery. **Results:** Our results demonstrated that intraluminal stenting significantly reduced the incidence of postoperative complications related to hypotony. Notably, no cases of choroidal detachment occurred in the nylon-stenting group (nsMS) compared to 30% (6 eyes) in the MS-only group (p = 0.0064). The hypotony rates between the nsMS (21.74%, 5 eyes) and the MS-only group (40%, 8 eyes) did not significantly differ (p = 0.3184). Both groups experienced significant reductions in intraocular pressure ($p < 0.001$) and a decrease in the number of antiglaucomatous medications ($p < 0.001$) up to four months after surgery. **Conclusions:** The use of an intraluminal stent (10.0 nylon suture) during MS implantation may be a promising strategy to reduce the risk of hypotony-related complications, particularly choroidal detachment, in patients with PEXG.

Keywords: glaucoma; pseudoexfoliation; MicroShunt; nylon stenting; hypotony

1. Introduction

PRESERFLO™ MicroShunt (MS) (Santen, Osaka, Japan) is a filtering procedure that is increasingly used to treat primary open-angle glaucoma (POAG). It is an 8.5 mm long synthetic polymer (SIBS—poly(styrene-block-isobutylene-block-styrene)) tube with a 70 μm diameter lumen, which after implantation allows fluid to flow directly from the anterior chamber of the eye to a filtering bleb underneath the conjunctiva [1]. It has been shown that MicroShunt (MS) effectively achieves low target intraocular pressure (IOP) levels in moderate to severe glaucoma, while reducing or eliminating the need for multiple glaucoma medications [1–4]. Compared to traditional filtering surgeries like trabeculectomy or glaucoma drainage devices (Ahmed Glaucoma Valve or Baerveldt Glaucoma Implant), MicroShunt (MS) is less invasive, poses a lower risk of complications, and has faster visual rehabilitation [1–3].

However, managing patients with pseudoexfoliation glaucoma (PEXG) presents considerable challenges. PEXG, characterized by the deposition of amyloid on the lens, iris, and trabecular meshwork, is often more aggressive and tends to progress rapidly. The extent of anatomical changes due to PEX can be assessed based on slit-lamp findings, like exfoliation load, angle involvement, and zonular instability [5–7]., whereas the severity of PEXG is commonly assessed using mean deviation (MD) from visual field testing. These anatomical changes are clinically relevant, as they could potentially influence surgical outcomes. Unfortunately, detailed grading of PEX severity was not available in our retrospective dataset. Due to these changes, PEXG patients are known to be more susceptible to postoperative complications, particularly intraocular hypotony [3,5]. This can subsequently result in severe conditions such as choroidal detachment, hypotony maculopathy, bleeding, and, in some cases, irreversible vision loss [3]. MicroShunt (MS) has been shown to be equally effective in lowering IOP and reducing glaucoma medication in patients with PEXG, with outcomes comparable to those in primary open-angle glaucoma (POAG) [8]. Furthermore, MicroShunt (MS) has been found to be non-inferior to trabeculectomy surgery (TET) in PEXG patients [3].

To minimize the risk of early postoperative hypotony and its complications, non-resorbable sutures can be used as intraluminal stents to ensure controlled drainage of aqueous humor and thus reduce the risk of excessively low IOP and complications such as choroidal detachment [9,10]. Beyond stabilizing IOP, intraluminal stenting also offers several additional benefits. By ensuring a steady, controlled flow of aqueous humor, it promotes proper healing around the shunt and reduces inflammation. Moreover, suture stents are easy to manage during surgery and can be removed at the slit lamp without the need for additional surgery [9,11,12].

This study aims to evaluate the impact of intraluminal stenting with a 10-0 nylon suture in patients with PEXG undergoing MicroShunt (MS) surgery.

The primary goal is to determine whether this technique reduces the incidence of postoperative hypotony and its complications, such as choroidal detachment and vision-threatening hypotony maculopathy. In addition, the study will assess the effect of intraluminal stenting on IOP control, IOP-lowering medication use, time to stent removal, treatment failure, visual acuity, visual field progression, and adverse events during the first four months after surgery.

2. Materials and Methods

2.1. Study Design

This was a single-center retrospective case-control study including all consecutive patients who underwent MicroShunt (MS) implantation with or without intraluminal stenting at the Department of Ophthalmology, LMU University Hospital, for uncontrolled PEXG between July 2019 and February 2020, and December 2023 and July 2024.

Clinical data was collected according to the principles of the Declaration of Helsinki and approved by the local regulatory ethics committee (Nr. 25-0296). Written informed consent was obtained from all patients.

2.2. Study Population

All participants were diagnosed with PEXG that was not adequately controlled with maximum tolerated medical therapy or was progressing despite treatment. Patients who were candidates for glaucoma surgery were eligible for inclusion.

Due to the occurrence of low postoperative IOP following MicroShunt (MS) surgery in patients with PEXG, intraluminal stenting of the MicroShunt (MS) using a 10-0 nylon suture was introduced as a modification. This retrospective analysis included patients who were divided into two groups based on the surgical technique: those who received MicroShunt (MS) implantation with a 10-0 nylon stent (nsMS group) and those who received MicroShunt (MS) without the stent (MS-only group). Due to the retrospective design of the study, there is a potential risk of selection bias, as the decision to use a stent was not randomized but based on individual clinical judgment. Only standalone procedures were performed.

2.3. Study Measurements

Postoperative visits followed a standardized regimen. Patients remained in the hospital for two days after surgery, with subsequent follow-up visits at intervals of one week to four weeks, six to eight weeks, and three to four months after surgery.

Before surgery, Visual Field 30-2 testing (Humphrey Field Analyzer 3; Carl Zeiss AG, Oberkochen, Germany) was conducted. Baseline demographic data (age, sex, lens status, spherical refraction, glaucoma medications) were also recorded. For each visit, the patients underwent a comprehensive ophthalmic evaluation, including slit lamp biomicroscopy, fundoscopy, and Goldmann applanation tonometry.

2.4. Surgical Success and Failure

In accordance with the World Glaucoma Association's Guidelines on the Design and Reporting of Glaucoma Surgical Trials [13], failure was defined by any of the following criteria:

1. IOP greater than 17 mmHg or less than 5 mmHg on two consecutive visits.
2. Less than 20% reduction in IOP from baseline on two consecutive visits.
3. The need for surgical revision or reoperation.
4. Loss of light perception.

The first and second postoperative days were excluded from the assessment of surgical success. Needling was not classified as a failure. Complete success was defined as meeting no failure criteria at four months without medication, while qualified success was defined as meeting no failure criteria at four months with medication.

2.5. PRESERFLO™ MicroShunt Implantation

MicroShunt (MS) implantation with or without stenting with a 10.0 suture was performed. Initially, a corneal traction suture was placed with 6-0 silk. A conjunctival limbal incision was made in the superonasal or superotemporal quadrant of the eye, Tenon's capsule and conjunctiva were dissected, and episcleral tissue was removed. Three sponges soaked in Mitomycin C 0.02% (0.2 mg/mL) were applied to the subtenon space for 2 min, then thoroughly rinsed with balanced salt solution. Afterwards, a 1 mm lance was used to create a scleral tunnel 3 mm from the limbus. A 25-gauge needle was then used to create a path between the iris and cornea, through which the MicroShunt (MS) was inserted in the anterior chamber. The MicroShunt (MS) was irrigated with balanced salt solution (BSS) to verify its function. Nylon stenting was carried out similarly to what has previously been described by Luke et al. [14]: One end of the nylon thread was inserted into the lumen of the MicroShunt (MS). An intrastromal corneal incision was made close to the limbus using a 15-degree knife. The other end of the nylon thread was then embedded in this corneal incision (Figure 1). This step was skipped in the control group. The conjunctiva and Tenon's capsule were finally placed over the shunt and attached to the limbus with 9-0 Vicryl sutures. A peribulbar injection of 4 mg dexamethasone was applied to reduce postoperative inflammation, followed by topical dexagentamicin ointment, and placement of an eye patch. The procedure was performed under local anesthesia (retrobulbar block) or general anesthesia.

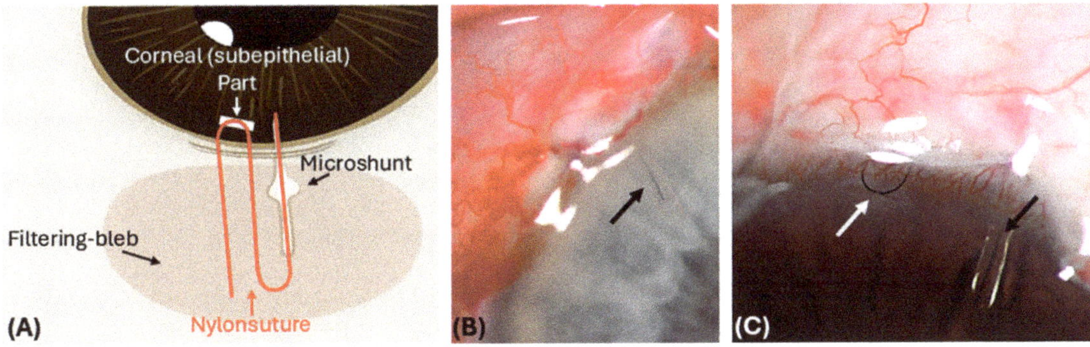

Figure 1. Postoperative (1 day) images showing the position of the 10.0 nylon suture inside the PreserFlo MicroShunt tube. (**A**) Schematic drawing of the placement of the 10.0 nylon suture inside the lumen and intracorneally (U-loop) (in red). (**B**) After implantation of the MicroShunt (MS) tube, a 10-0 nylon suture is advanced to the inner end of the tube (black arrow). (**C**) Then, a 10.0 nylon suture U-loop is embedded subepithelially in the area of the limbal cornea (white arrow), which enables easy postoperative access.

2.6. Post-Operative Management

2.6.1. Medication

Following surgery, a comprehensive care plan was implemented to ensure optimal healing and vision recovery. The specific treatment plan for each patient may vary based on individual factors such as IOP and bleb failure.

In general, postoperative management involved the following:

After surgery, the patients discontinued their previous glaucoma medications. To reduce inflammation and promote healing, a topical anti-inflammatory medication regimen (Prednisolone acetate 1% (10 mg/mL) eyedrops) was initiated. While first applied every hour, the dosage was then gradually tapered off every week. To prevent infection, a topical antibiotic (Levofloxacin eyedrops) was administered for a week.

The healing process, the state of the filtering bleb, and IOP were continuously monitored after surgery.

In case of low IOP (<5 mmHG) after surgery, atropine 0.5% eyedrops were started and continued until IOP was above 5 mmHG. IOP-lowering medications may be reintroduced or continued as necessary to maintain target IOP levels. The decision to adjust or discontinue these medications was made by the treating ophthalmologist based on the patient's individual needs and response to surgery.

2.6.2. Intraluminal Stent Removal

The criterion for stent removal was an IOP of over 15 mmHg. This criterion was based on the surgeons' clinical experience, aiming to balance the risk of early hypotony and high IOP values. The intraluminal stent removal was performed at the slit lamp under topical anesthesia by grasping the corneal end of the 10-0 nylon suture at the level of the cornea with forceps and pulling it out of the lumen.

2.6.3. Needling and Bleb Revision

Depending on the scarring of the bleb and IOP, 5-Fluorouracil (5-FU) was injected subconjunctivally near the bleb at the examiner's discretion. If bleb failure or other complications occurred, additional surgical interventions like needling or surgical revision were required. Needling and surgical revision were performed under sterile conditions in the operating room.

Needling was performed in cases of elevated IOP with a scarred and flat bleb. After topical anesthesia, lidocaine was injected under the conjunctiva near the bleb. A 30- or 27-gauge needle was then used to gently break down adhesions in the subconjunctival space both above and below the MicroShunt (MS) with controlled sweeping movements. Finally, 0.1 mL of 5-Fluorouracil (5-FU) was injected into the subconjunctival space, close to the bleb.

If needling failed to lower IOP or scarring in the bleb reappeared, surgical revision was performed. Tenon and conjunctiva were carefully dissected and scar tissue surrounding the implant was removed. Mitomycin C (0.02%; 0.2 mg/mL) was applied using a soaked sponge, which was left in place for two minutes. After removing the sponge, the eye and implant were thoroughly rinsed with BSS. The conjunctiva and Tenon's capsule were finally placed over the shunt and attached to the limbus with 9-0 Vicryl sutures. The procedure concluded with a peribulbar injection of 4 mg dexamethasone, topical dexagentamicin eyedrops, and an eye patch. Postoperative treatment followed the same protocol as after the initial implantation.

2.6.4. Outcome Measures

The primary outcome measure of the study is IOP and assessment of hypotony-related postoperative complications up to four months after surgery. Secondary outcome measures include the number of IOP-lowering medications and visual acuity, measured as best corrected visual acuity (BCVA) in Snellen. Snellen visual acuity measurements were converted to logMAR equivalents for analysis. Additional measures include the incidence of severe adverse events such as blebitis, endophthalmitis, corneal decompensation, retinal detachment, suprachoroidal hemorrhage, and wipe-out with complete vision loss.

2.6.5. Statistical Analysis

To evaluate potential associations between baseline demographic parameters and intraluminal stent use, multivariable regression analysis was performed with Bonferroni correction. Normal distribution of data was assessed using the Shapiro–Wilk test. Categorical variables like clinical and demographic data were presented as absolute numbers and percentages. Fisher's exact test was used for categorical variables, as appropriate. To compare means and proportions between the groups, Mann–Whitney U test was used as data was non-normally distributed. For a comparison of more than two groups, repeated measures ANOVA was used. Log-rank test was used to compare survival distributions. A post hoc power analysis was conducted to determine the minimum detectable effect size at a power of 0.8. A p-value of less than 0.05 was considered statistically significant. Confidence intervals (CIs) were calculated using a two-tailed method at a 95% confidence level. Statistical analyses and graph plotting were performed using Graphpad Prism for Windows (version 10.4.1; USA).

3. Results

3.1. Baseline Characteristics

This study included a total of 43 eyes, with 23 eyes in the MicroShunt with nylon stenting (nsMS) group and 20 eyes in the MicroShunt (MS-only) group. Baseline demographic data of both groups are presented in Table 1.

The patients ranged from 60 to 93 years old, with a median age of 75.7 ± 8.2 years. Both groups had similar age (p = 0.98, Mann–Whitney U test) and gender (p = 0.07, Fisher's exact test). Preoperative intraocular pressure (p = 0.3289, ANOVA) and BCVA (p = 0.3129, Mann–Whitney U test) were comparable between the two groups. The nsMS group showed greater visual field loss (mean deviation (MD) of the nsMS group was −14.66 decibel (dB) ± 9.28 dB, whereas mean MD of MS-only group was −7.65 dB ± 5.76 dB (p = 0.01, Mann–Whitney U test)).

Table 1. Summary of demographic characteristics of study patients at baseline in the MS-only and nsMS groups.

	nsMS (10.0) (n = 23)	MS-Only (n = 20)	p
Age (y, mean ± SD)	75.54 ± 7.79	75.95 ± 8.85	0.98 [a]
Female [n (%)]	8 (34.8%)	13 (65%)	0.0690 [b]
Pseudophakic [n (%)]	14 (60.9%)	15 (75%)	0.3528 [b]
Bilateral cases [(%)]	2 (9%)	2 (9%)	>0.9999 [b]
Combined surgery [(%)]	0 (0%)	1 (5%)	0.4651 [b]
Baseline IOP (mmHG)	23.54 ± 7.81	21.4 ± 5.76	0.3289 [c]
Baseline MD (mean ± SD)	−14.54 ± 9.38	−7.65 ± 5.76	0.01 [a]
Baseline BCVA (logmar, mean ± SD)	0.30 ± 0.22	0.18 ± 0.22	0.3129 [c]
Baseline medications (n, mean ± SD)	2.88 ± 1.19	2.75 ± 1.29	0.7919 [a]
CCT (μm, mean ± SD)	532.18 ± 37.17	544.7 ± 52.76	0.18 [a]

[a] Mann–Whitney U test; [b] Fisher's exact test; [c] repeated measures ANOVA; CCT = central cornea thickness; BCVA = best corrected visual acuity; MD = mean deviation, SD = standard deviation.

The same number and types of intraocular pressure-lowering medications were used by both groups preoperatively (p = 0.79, Mann–Whitney U test). Meanwhile, lens status (p = 0.35, Fisher's exact test), corneal thickness (p = 0.18, Mann–Whitney U test), spherical refraction (p = 0.91, Mann–Whitney U test), and the history of prior glaucoma surgeries ($p \geq 0.9999$ Fisher's exact test) were comparable.

Multivariable regression analysis found that among demographic factors, visual field loss, expressed as MD, was significantly associated with stent use (p = 0.007, Bonferroni-corrected multivariable regression analysis). Other factors, including age, sex, pseudophakia, baseline visual acuity, IOP, and number of medications, did not show statistically significant associations.

3.2. Primary Outcome Measures

At all measured timepoints up to 4 months (Figure 2), intraocular pressure (IOP) decreased significantly in the MS-only group from a preoperative mean of 21.4 mmHg (±5.76) [CI 95%: 18.70 to 24.10 mmHg] to postoperative means at each timepoint: 1 day (7.4 mmHg ± 3.8) [CI 95%: 5.64 to 9.16 mmHg], 2 days (7.05 mmHg ± 3.2) [CI 95%: 5.57 to 8.53 mmHg], 1–4 weeks (7.8 mmHg ± 3.4) [CI 95%: 6.18 to 9.35 mmHg], 6–8 weeks (9.6 mmHg ± 2.7) [CI 95%: 8.33 to 10.87 mmHg], and 3–4 months (10.81 mmHg ± 2.28) [CI 95%: 9.74 to 11.88 mmHg] ($p < 0.001$, Mann–Whitney U test).

Also, in the nsMS group, IOP declined from a preoperative mean of 23.54 mmHg (±7.81 mmHg) [CI 95%: 20.16 to 26.92 mmHg] to postoperative means at 1 day

(8.8 mmHg ± 3.8 mmHg) [CI 95%: 7.18 to 10.49 mmHg], 2 days (8.0 mmHg ± 3.5) [CI 95%: 6.50 to 9.50 mmHg], 1–4 weeks (10.6 mmHg ± 5.3) [CI 95%: 8.32 to 12.88 mmHg], 6–8 weeks (13.0 mmHg ± 8.5) [CI 95%: 9.28 to 16.62 mmHg], and 3–4 months (11.90 mmHg ± 5.01) [CI 95%: 9.74 to 14.07 mmHg]. This reduction was also statistically significant ($p < 0.001$, Mann–Whitney U test) (Figure 2).

After 4 months postoperatively, there was a reduction in the IOP of 49.45% in the nsMS group versus 49.49% in the MS-only group. The IOP reduction to preoperative values did not differ between the groups at all measured timepoints up to 4 months postoperatively. Significance levels are depicted in Figure 2. The achieved powers were calculated to be 0.23 (minimum effect size: 112) at day 1, 0.151 (minimum effect size: 192) at day 2, 0.546 (minimum effect size: 40) at week 1–4, 0.407 (minimum effect size: 58) at week 4–6, and 0.483 (minimum effect size: 47) at month 3–4.

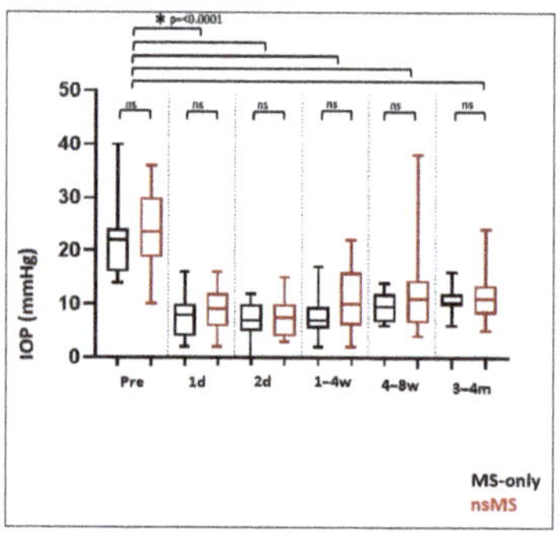

IOP (mmHg, mean ± SD)	nsMS	MS-only	p
pre-surgery	*23.5±7.8*	*21.4± 5.8*	*0.3289*
1d post-surgery	8.8±3.8	7.4± 3.8	0.3722
2d post-surgery	8.0±3.5	7.05 ± 3.2	0.5396
1–4w post-surgery	10.6±5.3	7.8 ±3.40	0.094
4–8w post-surgery	13.0±8.5	9.6 ±2.7	0.0866
3–4m post-surgery	11.9±5.0	10.8±2.3	0.4479

Figure 2. Development of IOP (mmHg) in the MS-only and nsMS groups from preoperative levels to the four-month follow-up visit (mean ± SD). IOP decreased significantly in both the MS-only and the nsMS group from before surgery to 4 months postoperatively ($p < 0.001$, Mann–Whitney U test). The reduction in IOP did not differ between the groups at all measured times up to 4 months postoperatively (d = day; w = week; m = month; ns = not significant).

The lowest recorded IOP was 0 mmHG in the MS-only group and 2 mmHg in the nsMS group. The rate of hypotony was higher in the MS-only group (40%) compared to the nsMS group (21.74%), though this difference did not show to be statistically significant ($p = 0.3184$, Mann–Whitney U test). Achieved power was 0.162 (minimum effect size: 110) (Figure 2).

3.3. Medical Therapy

In both groups, the average number of IOP-lowering medications significantly decreased in the nsMS group from 2.88 ± 1.19 to 0 ($p < 0.0001$; Fisher's exact test) and in the MS-only group from 2.75 ± 1.2 to 0.25 ($p < 0.0001$; Fisher's exact test) after 3 to 4 months. As illustrated in Figure 3, after 3 months, a single eye (4.3%) in the nsMS group needed three IOP-lowering drugs within 4 to 8 weeks. This eye received needling after a week and bleb revision after 2 weeks post-surgery due to bleb failure. IOP-lowering medication was no longer indicated after these procedures.

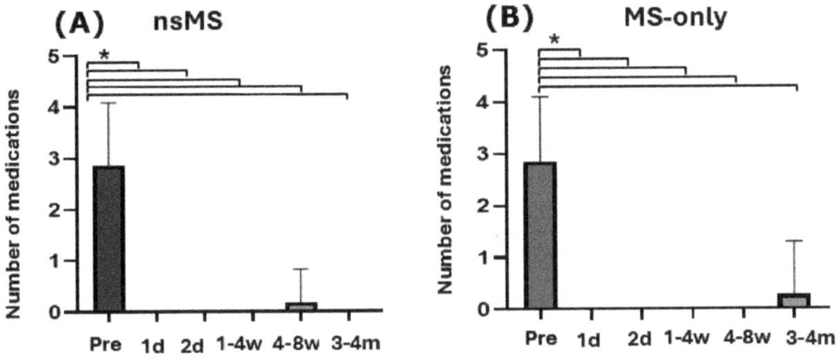

Figure 3. Histogram showing the number of IOP-lowering medications used preoperatively from day 1 to the 4-month follow-up visit (mean ± SD). In both groups, the average number of IOP-lowering medications significantly decreased after 3 to 4 months. (**A**) In the nsMS group antiglaucomatous medication decreased from 2.88 ± 1.19 to 0 ($p < 0.0001$; Fisher's exact test) (**B**) In the MS-only group antiglaucomatous medication decreased from 2.75 ± 1.2 to 0.25 ($p < 0.0001$; Fisher's exact test) (Pre = preoperatively; d = day; w = week; m = month; * $p \leq 0.0001$)).

In the MS-only group, one eye (5%) needed 4 IOP-lowering eyedrops after 4 months, because of progressive visual field defects despite an IOP of 13 mmHG.

There was no significant difference in reduction of medication between the two groups ($p \geq 0.9999$; Fisher's exact test). The calculated power for this comparison was 0.062 (minimum effect size: 156).

3.4. Intraluminal Stenting

In 14 eyes (60.87%), the intraluminal stent was removed, with an average removal time of 52.72 ± 40.45 days [CI 95%: 29.35 to 76.09 days] (Figure 4) and a mean IOP reduction of 4.19 ± 3.6 mmHg [CI 95%: 2.11 to 6.27 mmHg] after removal. Pre-removal IOP was 18.86 ± 5.72 mmHg [CI 95%: 15.56 to 22.16 mmHg], dropping to 14.67 ± 9.31 mmHg [CI 95%: 9.29 to 20.05 mmHg] ($p = 0.038$, Mann–Whitney U test) (Figure 4).

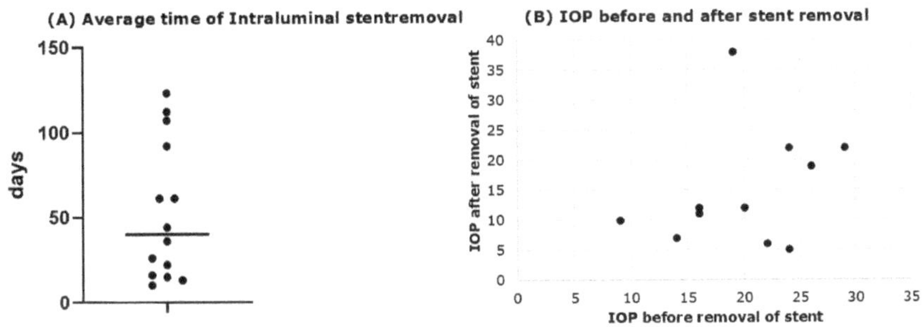

Figure 4. Time of stent removal and effect on IOP. (**A**) Average removal time of intraluminal stent (average removal time of 52.72 ± 40.45 days); (**B**) IOP before and after stent removal. Pre-removal IOP was 18.86 ± 5.72 mmHg, dropping to 14.67 ± 9.31 mmHg ($p = 0.03836$, Mann–Whitney U test).

3.5. Postoperative Complications

Table 2 provides an overview of the postoperative complications in each group. The most prevalent complication was hypotony. Hypotony occurred in 21.74% eyes in the nsMS group (5 eyes) and 40% in the MS-only group (8 eyes), with no statistically significant difference ($p = 0.3184$; Fisher's exact test). The power reached was calculated to be 0.162

(minimum effect size: 110). All cases of hypotony in the MS-only group occurred early after surgery and resolved within the first 6 weeks. In six eyes in the MS-only group and in one case in the nsMS group, hypotony resolved spontaneously. Others required conservative treatment with topical atropine and/or therapeutic contact lenses (four eyes (80%) in the nsMS group and two eyes (10%) in the MS-only group). In total, 2 cases (10%) in the MS-only group and 0 cases (0%) in the nsMS group required stabilization of the anterior chamber with viscoelastic.

However, the MS-only group experienced significantly more complications related to excessively low IOP. Specifically, 6 eyes (30%) in the MS group without nylon stenting developed choroidal detachment. In contrast, none (0%) of the patients in the nsMS group experienced these complications ($p = 0.0064$, Fisher's exact test). Achieved power was 0.752 (minimum effect size: 24). Interestingly, five days after removal of the intraluminal stent, one patient experienced intraocular hypotony with choroidal detachment; however, the intraocular hypotony and choroidal detachment resolved spontaneously after the use of topical atropine 1%.

Both groups experienced complications such as Seidel-positive leakage (one in the MS-only group and two in the nsMS group ($p \geq 0.9999$, Fisher's exact test)) and a flat anterior chamber (three in the MS-only group and one in the nsMS group ($p = 0.3235$, Fisher's exact test)). Hyphema was seen in the MS-only group in 4 cases, but nsMS did not experience hyphema ($p = 0.0393$, Fisher's exact test)

Table 2. Postoperative complications after MS-only and nsMS surgery.

	nsMS ($n = 23$)	MS-Only ($n = 20$)	p
Hypotony (in%)	5 (21.74%)	8 (40%)	0.3184
Choroidal detachment (in%)	(0) 0%	(6) 30%	0.0064
Flat anterior chamber (n (%))	(1) 4%	(3) 15%	0.3235
Macular folds	(0) 0%	(0) 0%	
Hyphema	(0) 0%	(4) 20%	0.0393
Corneal complications (n (%))	(1) 4%	(3) 15%	0.3235
Corneal dellen (n (%))	(0) 0%	(0) 0%	>0.9999
Corneal erosion (n (%))	(0) 0%	(2) 10%	0.2104
Corneal edema (n (%))	(1) 4%	(1) 5%	>0.9999
Seidel positive (n (%))	(2; Seidel I + Seidel II) 9%	(1; Seidel I) 5%	>0.9999
Implant extrusion (n (%))	0%	(0) 0%	>0.9999
Blebitis (n (%))	0%	(0) 0%	>0.9999
Loss of light perception (n (%))	0%	(0) 0%	>0.9999

Data are presented as numbers and percentages of the total number for the respective treatment group (MS-only or nsMS). The nsMS group had significantly lower number of choroidal detachment ($p = 0.0064$, Fisher's exact test) and hyphema ($p = 0.0393$, Fisher's exact test). Other complications were similar.

Corneal erosion could be observed in two patients in the MS-only group, whereas it was absent in the nsMS group ($p = 0.2104$, Fisher's exact test). Both groups experienced one case of corneal edema ($p \geq 0.9999$, Fisher's exact test). In none of the groups, macular folds, corneal dellen, implant extrusion, blebitis, or loss of light perception was recorded.

Importantly, no serious adverse events were reported in either group.

The resulting power was calculated to be 0.51 (minimum effect size: 676) for Seidel-positive leakage, 0.111 (minimum effect size: 121) for flat anterior chamber, 0.458 for hyphema (minimum effect size: 37), 0.135 (minimum effect size: 76) for corneal erosion, and 0.093 (minimum effect size: 692) for corneal edema.

3.6. Subconjunctival Injection of 5-FU, Needling, and Surgical Revision

In the MS-only group, subconjunctival 5-FU injections were administered 24 times (1.2 injections per case) compared to 40 times (1.74 injections per case) in the nsMS group ($p = 0.1004$, Fisher's exact test). The number of 5-FU injections did not differ significantly ($p = 0.117$, Fisher's exact test) between the two groups. The statistical power obtained was 0.170 (minimum effect size: 50).

A single 5-FU injection was sufficient in 11 cases (55%) in the MS-only group and 8 cases (34.78%) in the nsMS group. Two injections were required in 6 cases (30%) in the MS-only group and 12 cases (52.2%) in the nsMS group. Three injections were necessary in 3 cases (13.04%) in the nsMS group. Notably, 3 eyes (15%) in the MS group did not require any postoperative 5-FU injections, whereas every eye in the nsMS group received at least one.

On the second day and the 4- to 8-week mark, the total number of eyes requiring 5-FU injections differed significantly between the groups ($p = 0.0387$ and $p = 0.050$, Fisher's exact test), with the nsMS group receiving more injections. No significant differences could be observed at other timepoints ($p \geq 0.9999$, Fisher's exact test).

Needling was performed when a flat bleb, elevated IOP, or a Tenon's cyst were present. The total number of eyes requiring needling did not differ significantly between the two groups ($p > 0.9999$, Fisher's exact test). The calculated power was 0.067 (minimum effect size: 801). At all times, there was no significant difference in needling rates ($p > 0.9999$, Fisher's exact test).

Early bleb encapsulation requiring needling occurred in 2 cases (10%) in the MS-only group and 2 cases (8.7%) in the nsMS group. In the MS-only group, needling was performed at either day 1 or between 4 and 8 weeks postoperatively. In the nsMS group, needling was performed between 4 and 8 weeks and 3 and 4 months postoperatively.

Within the first week after surgery, two patients in the MS-only group required three interventions (three anterior chamber reformations with Healon (hyaluronic acid sodium 8.5 mg/0.85 mL)), while one patient in the nsMS group required a single intervention (re-suturing of the conjunctiva) ($p = 0.3475$, Fisher's exact test).

During the four-month follow-up, surgical revision was not needed in the MS-only group (0%), whereas it was necessary in three cases in the nsMS group (13%) ($p = 0.2464$, Fisher's exact test). Besides, one patient in the MS-only group required rescue surgery with repositioning and suture-fixation of the implant, along with occlusion of the tube using an 8.0 Ethilon suture. Whereas no such procedure was needed in the nsMS group ($p = 0.4773$, Fisher's exact test).

Further glaucoma surgery was required for one patient in the MS-only group. Four months after initial, complicated surgery and the above-mentioned rescue surgery on the fourth postoperative day as well as unsuccessful needling, cyclophotocoagulation was performed due to scarring of the bleb and conjunctiva as well as underlying systemic comorbitities that limited the feasibility of further glaucoma-valve surgery. Up to the four-month follow-up, no patients in the nsMS group required further surgery ($p = 0.4773$, Fisher's exact test).

3.7. Success Rates

In the MS-only group, 85% (17/20) achieved complete success compared to 65.3% (15/23) in the nsMS group ($p = 0.1396$; Log-rank test). Qualified success was achieved in 90% (18/20) of the MS-only group and 82.6% (19/23) of the nsMS group ($p = 0.1396$; log-rank test). Kaplan–Meier survival curves for complete success are shown in Figure 5.

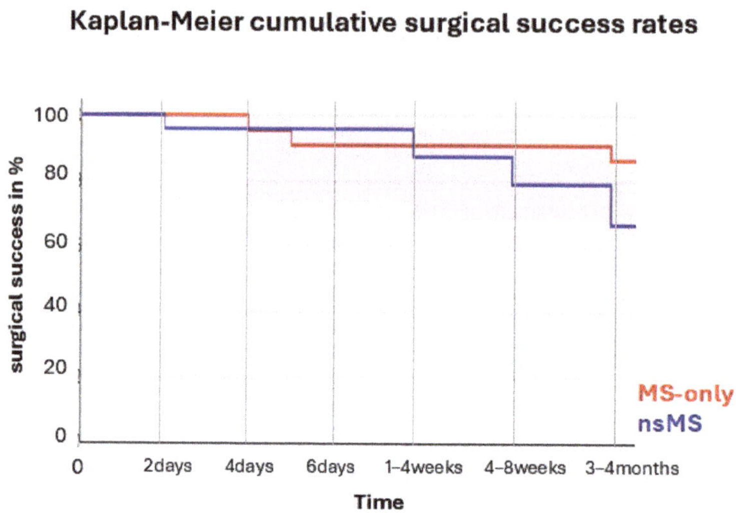

Figure 5. Kaplan–Meier survival curve of cumulative surgical success through four months of follow-up.

In the nsMS group, three patients (13.0%) experienced an IOP outside the 5–17 mmHg range on two consecutive visits—two after 3–4 months and one after 6 weeks. Moreover, another patient (4.3%) experienced an IOP reduction of less than 20% from baseline to 3–4 months compared to none in the MS-only group.

After four or five days, two patients (10%) in the MS-only group developed postoperative hypotony, requiring AC reformation with Healon. Another patient needed further glaucoma surgery (cyclophotokoagulation) after 4 months. In the nsMS group, one patient required surgery after 2 days (re-suturing of the conjunctiva) due to a Seidel I-positive filtering bleb and three patients required open revision surgery for a scarred bleb after two, four, and seven weeks (13.0%).

4. Discussion

Postoperative hypotony is a recognized risk for MicroShunt (MS) surgery. Unlike the Ahmed valve, which regulates aqueous outflow through a built-in resistance mechanism, MicroShunt (MS) is based on the principles of the Hagen–Poiseuille law and the gradual development of outflow resistance caused by fibrosis in the conjunctiva and Tenon's capsule [15,16]. This risk, along with the potential for sight-threatening complications such as choroidal detachment, macular folds, and suprachoroidal hemorrhage, is further heightened in PEXG patients undergoing MicroShunt (MS) surgery [3,16,17], as in PEXG patients, conjunctival and scleral healing can be impaired by oxidative stress and chronic inflammation due to exfoliative material [17,18]. Additionally, a higher incidence of complications such as zonular dialysis and vitreous loss may further disrupt drainage through the MicroShunt (MS) tube [5,19]. Consequently, to prevent hypotony in PEXG patients, measures like reducing outflow from the MicroShunt (MS) tube using a nylon stent should be considered during surgery.

This retrospective study of 43 eyes investigated the incidence of intraocular hypotony in patients with PEX glaucoma undergoing MicroShunt (MS) implantation with (n = 23) or without (n = 20) intraluminal stenting with a 10.0 nylon suture. The follow-up period was 4 months after surgery. Although the use of a 10.0 nylon stent for outflow restriction as a treatment for prolonged postoperative hypotony has been described previously [10–12], this, to our knowledge, is the first study to evaluate the efficacy of MicroShunt (MS) flow restriction in PEX glaucoma eyes and its preventive impact on early hypotony rates and associated complications. The two groups were demographically comparable, except for significantly more advanced visual field defects (expressed as mean deviation (MD)) in the nsMS group ($p = 0.01$). Moreover, MD significantly predicted the likelihood of stent implantation ($p = 0.007$). This may be attributed to consistent clinical outcomes with MicroShunt (MS) implantation in PEXG cases, which has encouraged its use in more advanced stages of PEXG. However, it also suggests a potential treatment bias, whereby surgeons may have been more inclined to select patients with more severe disease for intraluminal stenting.

Previously, it was demonstrated that MicroShunt (MS) implantation is effective for PEXG, showing non-inferiority compared to trabeculectomy (TET) [3]. However, PEXG patients experienced a higher incidence of hypotony, particularly with anterior chamber shallowing, compared to MicroShunt (MS) surgery performed in patients with primary open-angle glaucoma (POAG) [8,20]. As a preventive measure, intraluminal stents may be used—similar to Baerveldt or Paul glaucoma drainage devices, where such stents are routinely placed and typically removed after 4 to 6 weeks.

Nylon stenting with a 10.0 nylon suture (20 μm diameter) reduces the lumen of the MS (70 μm diameter) by 29% and consequently decreases outflow. That is why lower rates of hypotony were hypothesized in the nsMS group, as demonstrated previously in other cohorts [10–12,14].

However, in the present study, no significant difference in early postoperative hypotony rates between the MS-only and nsMS groups could be found. Although the hypotony rate was higher in the MS-only group (40%, 8 eyes) compared to the nsMS group (21.74%, 5 eyes), the difference was not statistically significant ($p = 0.3184$). This lack of difference may be attributed to factors such as the extent of MicroShunt (MS) occlusion or the small sample size, causing this study to be underpowered to rule out a clinically meaningful difference. Moreover, in contrast to Luke et al., Lupardi et al., Miura et al., and Verma-Fuehring et al. [10–12,14], our patient population consisted solely of PEXG patients, who might respond differently to intraluminal stenting. PEXG is known to exhibit fluctuating IOP values and is generally more aggressive, with a higher risk of postoperative hypotony [17]. As mentioned before, the size of the suture could play a role in IOP control. Here, we used a 10.0 nylon suture, which is about 20 μm in diameter and occludes approximately 29% of the MicroShunt (MS) (lumen: 70 μm diameter). In contrast, Luke et al. [14] used a thicker 8-0 polyamide suture, which has a larger diameter (40 μm) and occludes up to 50% of the MicroShunt (MS) lumen. The thicker suture may be more effective in reducing postoperative hypotony. However, it is important to distinguish uncomplicated hypotony—which typically resolves spontaneously within 4–6 weeks—from clinical hypotony associated with complications such as choroidal detachment and anterior chamber shallowing.

Although the overall difference in the rate of hypotony did not reach statistical significance, clinical hypotony was significantly lower in the nsMS group. Notably, no cases of choroidal detachment, a serious sight-threatening complication, occurred in the stenting group compared to 30% (6 eyes) in the MS-only group ($p = 0.0064$). Interestingly, hyphema occurred less frequently in the nsMS group ($p = 0.0393$), possibly due to a lower incidence of clinical hypotony, as reflux bleeding is associated with excessively low postoperative IOP levels. Other complications, such as corneal edema ($p > 0.9999$), corneal erosion ($p = 0.2104$), and shallow anterior chamber ($p = 0.3235$), remained comparable between the groups. This could suggest that nylon stenting does not cause additional trauma.

While the intraluminal stent provided fewer hypotony-related complications, it did not significantly affect long-term IOP control or the need for glaucoma medications. Both groups had comparable reductions in anti-glaucoma eyedrop usage ($p = 0.999$), and surgical success ($p = 0.1396$) was similar. Needling rates in our study were the same in both groups (Needling: MS-only group 10% and nsMS-group 8.7%) and in line with previously published studies. Thus, needling rates of 5% to 19% were reported after one year of follow-up [14,21]. Additionally, the number of eyes ($p = 0.117$) needing 5-FU injections and total number of 5-FU injections did not differ significantly ($p = 0.10$). These findings suggest that the 10.0 intraluminal stent appears to effectively stabilize IOP without compromising MicroShunt (MS) filtration efficacy at up to 4 months.

However, four patients in the nsMS group experienced IOP levels greater than 17 mmHg or a reduction of less than 20%. This could be attributed to the intraluminal stent not yet being removed; therefore, optimal timing for stent removal is essential to achieve better long-term IOP control. Nevertheless, to avoid hypotony after early suture removal, we recommend pulling out the nylon suture no earlier than 4 weeks, once the drainage bleb has formed. If necessary, in the case of rising IOP, topical anti-glaucoma medications, preferably beta-blockers or carbonic anhydrase inhibitors, should be used during this period. In cases where IOP remains consistently below 15 mmHg, the intraluminal stent is retained long-term. This approach is based on findings from previous studies [10–12,14], which have not demonstrated any disadvantages associated with stent retention. Maintaining the stent could help reduce the risk of delayed-onset hypotony, which can occur even after initially stable postoperative outcomes. However, a longer follow-up period would be required to thoroughly assess the long-term safety and efficacy of this approach.

However, patients with nylon stenting may be at an increased risk of complications, such as endophthalmitis. This risk is thought to arise from the stent serving as a conduit between the anterior chamber and the subconjunctival space [12,22]. None of our patients experienced this complication, and moreover, previous studies have reported no cases of infection following intraluminal stent placement [10–12,14]. To minimize the risk of infection, we adopted a technique first described by Luke et al. [14], in which the nylon suture is embedded into the cornea (Figure 1). Burying the external end of the suture in a corneal groove simplifies postoperative management, lowers the risk of bacterial invasion, reduces the need for invasive removal procedures, minimizes accidental suture pullout, and improves patient comfort.

In conclusion, this study provides preliminary evidence that intraluminal stenting with a 10.0 nylon suture during MicroShunt (MS) implantation may be a promising strategy to reduce the risk of hypotony-related complications in PEXG patients. The technique is minimally invasive and technically straightforward and integrates seamlessly into existing surgical workflows. However, this study has several limitations. Its retrospective design may introduce selection bias and limit control over data collection, as the decision to use a stent may have been influenced by clinical judgment, potentially favoring stent placement in higher-risk cases. Indeed, glaucoma severity, as measured by mean MD, was significantly associated with stent implantation ($p = 0.007$), suggesting a possible treatment bias in which surgeons preferentially selected patients with more advanced PEXG for intraluminal stenting. This bias may confound interpretation of treatment outcomes, as more severe baseline disease could lead to different postoperative trajectories. Glaucoma severity was assessed using visual field MD as recommended by the World Glaucoma Association's

Guidelines on the Design and Reporting of Glaucoma Surgical Trials. However, we did not apply a PEX-specific grading system that considers factors such as exfoliation load, angle involvement, or zonular instability. This limits our ability to address disease heterogeneity within the PEXG population. Prospective studies with standardized criteria for stent selection are needed to reduce bias and more accurately assess the efficacy of stenting across varying disease severities.

Lastly, the relatively small sample size (n = 43) limits the statistical power and generalizability of our findings. Several comparisons did not reach statistical significance and should therefore be interpreted with caution. Post hoc power analysis indicated insufficient power to detect small to moderate effect sizes, meaning that the study may not have been adequately powered to rule out clinically relevant differences. Larger, well-powered studies are warranted to validate and expand upon these results.

Author Contributions: Conceptualization: M.J.M. and L.F.K.; Interventions: M.J.M., L.F.K. and S.G.P.; Data curation: M.G.; Formal analysis: M.G.; Writing—original draft: M.G.; Writing—review and editing: M.J.M., L.F.K. and L.B.; Visualization: M.G.; Project administration: L.F.K.; Funding acquisition: M.J.M. All authors have read and agreed to the published version of the manuscript.

Funding: An intramural funding was granted to Dr Keidel (Munich Medical & Clinician Scientist Program, LMU Munich; https://www.med.lmu.de/karriere/mcsp/index.html (accessed on 1 July 2023), funding number CS051). Research funding or study-related expenses were provided by Iridex and iSTAR Medical.

Institutional Review Board Statement: The collection of clinical data was conducted according to the principles of the Declaration of Helsinki and was given local regulatory approval by the ethics committee (Nr. 25-0296; 12 June 2025).

Informed Consent Statement: Written informed consent was obtained from all patients prior to their planned surgical procedures.

Data Availability Statement: All relevant data was provided in the manuscript.

Conflicts of Interest: Miranda Gehrke and Lara Buhl declare no conflicts of Interest. The funder played no role in study design, data collection, analysis and interpretation of the data or the writing of this manuscript. Leonie Keidel has received speaker fees and/or travel expenses from Alcon Pharma GmbH, Novartis Pharma GmbH, Recordati Rare Diseases Inc., CHIESI GmbH, Roche Diagnostics GmbH, DORC Holding BV, and Santen GmbH. Siegfried Priglinger has received speaker fees and/or travel expenses from Novartis Pharma GmbH, Oertli AG, Bayer AG, Alcon Pharma GmbH, and Pharm-Allergan GmbH. Marc Mackert has received speaker fees from iSTAR Medical, Sight Sciences, Santen GmbH, and AbbVie. Marc Mackert has also received support for attending meetings from Alcon Pharma GmbH, AbbVie, and iSTAR Medical. The funders had no role in the design of the study; in the collection, analyses, or interpretation of data; in the writing of the manuscript; or in the decision to publish the results. None of the authors' financial interests are directly or indirectly related to this work.

References

1. Saeed, E.; Golaszewska, K.; Dmuchowska, D.A.; Zalewska, R.; Konopinska, J. The PreserFlo MicroShunt in the Context of Minimally Invasive Glaucoma Surgery: A Narrative Review. *Int. J. Environ. Res. Public Health* **2023**, *20*, 2904. [CrossRef] [PubMed] [PubMed Central]
2. Scheres, L.M.J.; van den Biggelaar, F.; Winkens, B.; Kujovic-Aleksov, S.; Muskens, R.; de Waard, P.W.T.; de Crom, R.M.P.C.; Ernest, P.J.G.; Pijl, B.J.; Ramdas, W.D.; et al. Effectiveness and cost-effectiveness of MicroShunt implantation versus standard trabeculectomy for open-angle glaucoma (a SIGHT study): Study protocol of a multicentre randomised controlled trial. *BMC Ophthalmol.* **2023**, *23*, 43. [CrossRef] [PubMed] [PubMed Central]

3. Nobl, M.; Grun, C.; Kassumeh, S.; Priglinger, S.; Mackert, M.J. One-Year Outcomes of Preserflo(TM) MicroShunt Implantation versus Trabeculectomy for Pseudoexfoliation Glaucoma. *J. Clin. Med.* **2023**, *12*, 3000. [CrossRef] [PubMed] [PubMed Central]
4. Storp, J.J.; Vietmeier, F.E.; Merté, R.L.; Koch, R.; Zimmermann, J.A.; Eter, N.; Brücher, V.C. Long-Term Outcomes of the PRESERFLO MicroShunt Implant in a Heterogeneous Glaucoma Cohort. *J. Clin. Med.* **2023**, *12*, 4474. [CrossRef] [PubMed] [PubMed Central]
5. Plateroti, P.; Plateroti, A.M.; Abdolrahimzadeh, S.; Scuderi, G. Pseudoexfoliation Syndrome and Pseudoexfoliation Glaucoma: A Review of the Literature with Updates on Surgical Management. *J. Ophthalmol.* **2015**, *2015*, 370371. [CrossRef] [PubMed] [PubMed Central]
6. Yuksel, N.; Yilmaz Tugan, B. Pseudoexfoliation Glaucoma: Clinical Presentation and Therapeutic Options. *Turk. J. Ophthalmol.* **2023**, *53*, 247–256. [CrossRef] [PubMed] [PubMed Central]
7. Nobl, M.; Mackert, M. Pseudoexfoliation Syndrome and Glaucoma. *Klin. Monbl. Augenheilkd.* **2019**, *236*, 1139–1155. [CrossRef] [PubMed]
8. Nobl, M.; Freissinger, S.; Kassumeh, S.; Priglinger, S.; Mackert, M.J. One-year outcomes of microshunt implantation in pseudoexfoliation glaucoma. *PLoS ONE* **2021**, *16*, e0256670. [CrossRef] [PubMed] [PubMed Central]
9. Aguilar-Munoa, S.; Tham, Y.H.; Barton, K. A simple surgical solution for the treatment of persistent postoperative hypotony after PRESERFLO MicroShunt implantation. *Eye* **2023**, *37*, 2126–2129. [CrossRef] [PubMed] [PubMed Central]
10. Verma-Fuehring, R.; Dakroub, M.; Bamousa, A.; Kann, G.; Hillenkamp, J.; Kampik, D. The use of intraluminal PRESERFLO stenting in avoiding early postoperative hypotony. *Graefes Arch. Clin. Exp. Ophthalmol.* **2024**, *262*, 3925–3932. [CrossRef] [PubMed] [PubMed Central]
11. Miura, Y.; Fukuda, K.; Yamashiro, K. Comparison of outcomes with and without intrastent placement during PMS surgery. *Sci. Rep.* **2025**, *15*, 2981. [CrossRef] [PubMed]
12. Lupardi, E.; Laffi, G.L.; Moramarco, A.; Barboni, P.; Fontana, L. Systematic Preserflo MicroShunt Intraluminal Stenting for Hypotony Prevention in Highly Myopic Patients: A Comparative Study. *J. Clin. Med.* **2023**, *12*, 1677. [CrossRef] [PubMed] [PubMed Central]
13. Shaarawy, T.; Grehn, F.; Sherwood, M.; World Glaucoma, A. *WGA Guidelines on Design and Reporting of Glaucoma Surgical Trials*, 1st ed.; Kugler Publications: The Hague, The Netherlands, 2009.
14. Luke, J.N.; Reinking, N.; Dietlein, T.S.; Haendel, A.; Enders, P.; Lappas, A. Intraoperative primary partial occlusion of the PreserFlo MicroShunt to prevent initial postoperative hypotony. *Int. Ophthalmol.* **2023**, *43*, 2643–2651. [CrossRef] [PubMed] [PubMed Central]
15. Budenz, D.L.; Barton, K.; Gedde, S.J.; Feuer, W.J.; Schiffman, J.; Costa, V.P.; Godfrey, D.G.; Buys, Y.M. Five-year treatment outcomes in the Ahmed Baerveldt comparison study. *Ophthalmology* **2015**, *122*, 308–316. [CrossRef] [PubMed] [PubMed Central]
16. Pereira, I.C.F.; Wyss, H.M.; Pinchuk, L.; Beckers, H.J.M.; den Toonder, J.M.J. A model for designing intraocular pressure-regulating glaucoma implants. *PLoS ONE* **2022**, *17*, e0273672. [CrossRef] [PubMed] [PubMed Central]
17. Drolsum, L.; Ringvold, A.; Nicolaissen, B. Cataract and glaucoma surgery in pseudoexfoliation syndrome: A review. *Acta Ophthalmol. Scand.* **2007**, *85*, 810–821. [CrossRef] [PubMed]
18. Borjan, I.; Stanić, R.; Pleština-Borjan, I.; Pavić, M.; Hertzberg, S.N.W.; Znaor, L.; Petrovski, B.É.; Petrovski, G. Pseudoexfoliative Syndrome in Cataract Surgery-A Quality Register Study and Health Economic Analysis in the Split-Dalmatia County, Croatia. *J. Clin. Med.* **2023**, *13*, 38. [CrossRef] [PubMed] [PubMed Central]
19. Tuteja, S.; Zeppieri, M.; Chawla, H. Pseudoexfoliation Syndrome and Glaucoma. In *StatPearls*; StatPearls Publishing Copyright © 2025; StatPearls Publishing LLC: Treasure Island, FL, USA, 2025.
20. Nobl, M.; Freissinger, S.; Rudolph, K.; Vounotrypidis, E.; Kassumeh, S.; Priglinger, S.; Mackert, M.J. Long-term Outcomes of PreserFlo MicroShunt versus XEN45 Gel Stent in Open-Angle Glaucoma. *Klin. Monbl Augenheilkd.* **2024**, *241*, 805–812. [CrossRef] [PubMed]
21. Bhayani, R.; Martinez de la Casa, J.M.; Figus, M.; Klabe, K.; Rabiolo, A.; Mercieca, K. Short-term safety and efficacy of Preserflo Microshunt in glaucoma patients: A multicentre retrospective cohort study. *Eye* **2023**, *37*, 644–649. [CrossRef] [PubMed] [PubMed Central]
22. Weber, C.; Herwig-Carl, M.C.; Holz, F.G.; Mercieca, K. Occlusion of the PreserFlo(R) MicroShunt implant by iris tissue. *Ophthalmologie* **2024**, *121*, 579–583. [CrossRef] [PubMed]

Journal of
Clinical Medicine

Article

Surgical Outcomes of XEN45 Gel Stent Using Ab Interno Technique in Open-Angle Glaucoma: A 2-Year Follow-Up Study

Doah Kim [1], Myungjin Kim [1], Marvin Lee [2] and Seungsoo Rho [1,*]

[1] Department of Ophthalmology, CHA Bundang Medical Center, CHA University, Seongnam 13496, Gyeonggi-do, Republic of Korea; inhamed93216006@gmail.com (D.K.); brandmjeyes@gmail.com (M.K.)
[2] Allbarun Eye Clinic, Suwon 16499, Gyeonggi-do, Republic of Korea; mvdevil@naver.com
* Correspondence: harryrho@gmail.com; Tel.: +82-780-1905

Abstract: Background/Objectives: This study aims to evaluate the long-term efficacy and safety of ab interno techniques using minimally invasive glaucoma surgery (MIGS), specifically XEN gel stent implantation, by evaluating its 2-year outcomes in patients with primary open-angle glaucoma (POAG) and pseudoexfoliation glaucoma (PXG). **Methods**: This retrospective single-center study consecutively included 31 eyes of 31 patients with POAG or PXG who underwent XEN gel stent implantation. Patients were followed for 24 months, with assessments at multiple time points. Success was defined as achieving an IOP of less than 14 mmHg and a reduction of more than 20% from preoperative IOP without additional glaucoma surgery. Bleb morphology was evaluated using anterior segment optical coherence tomography (AS-OCT) and slit-lamp photographs. Postoperative interventions and complications were also recorded. **Results**: At 24 months, complete success and qualified success rates were 35.5% (11/31) and 51.6% (16/31), respectively. There was no difference in surgical success rates at 2 years based on the tip location (intraconjunctiva, intratenon, and uviform) on the 1st postoperative day. Patients with high sparse wall on AS-OCT imaging or avascular bleb morphology via slit-lamp photography at 6 months postoperatively had higher complete success rates at 2 years than those without ($p = 0.007$, $p = 0.009$, respectively). Patients with avascular bleb types at 6 months postoperatively had higher qualified success rates at 2 years compared with the vascular types ($p = 0.038$). Needling was performed in 32.3% of eyes, with secondary surgical procedures required in 16.1% of eyes. The most common adverse event was hypotony, occurring in 67.7% of eyes on the 1st postoperative day but resolving within 6 months. **Conclusions**: The ab interno XEN gel stent is an effective and minimally invasive option for managing POAG and PXG, with long-term success predicted by the AS-OCT assessment of bleb morphology at 6 months. Proactive postoperative management, emphasizing early intervention and monitoring, is crucial for maintaining optimal outcomes.

Keywords: ab interno; bleb; intraocular pressure; MIGS; minimally invasive glaucoma surgery; open-angle glaucoma; XEN gel stent

1. Introduction

Ab interno techniques in minimally invasive glaucoma surgery (MIGS) have transformed the landscape of glaucoma management by offering less invasive alternatives to traditional filtration surgeries like trabeculectomy and glaucoma drainage devices (GDDs) for patients with early to moderate glaucoma [1,2]. These traditional surgeries are associated with high complication rates, prompting the widespread adoption of MIGS procedures in recent years, particularly in the United States from 2013 to 2018 [3].

Among the array of MIGS procedures available, the XEN gel stent (Allergan, Dublin, CA, USA) has emerged as a notable option. Designed for ab interno placement, the XEN gel stent acts as a subconjunctival drainage device, effectively lowering intraocular pressure (IOP) while demonstrating safety and efficacy profiles comparable to trabeculectomy [4,5]. The ab interno approach minimizes surgical trauma, reduces postoperative complications such as hyphema, and preserves corneal endothelial integrity [6–8]. By sparing the conjunctiva from extensive manipulation, this technique aims to prevent subconjunctival bleeding and enhance the physiological absorption of aqueous humor through preserved conjunctival lymphatics.

Studies have shown that the XEN gel stent effectively reduces IOP and medication burden in patients with primary open-angle glaucoma (POAG) and pseudoexfoliation glaucoma (PXG) [9–11]. Comparable outcomes have been reported for both standalone XEN procedures and those combined with cataract surgery in several studies [12–14]. Compared with traditional filtering surgeries such as trabeculectomy, the XEN gel stent offers a favorable safety profile with a lower incidence of complications [15,16]. In addition, bleb morphology evaluated by anterior segment OCT has been proposed as a meaningful predictor of long-term surgical success [17,18].

In our previous study, we conducted a 6-month follow-up on patients who underwent XEN gel stent implantation and identified key predictors of surgical success by evaluating clinical parameters and bleb morphology using anterior segment optical coherence tomography (AS-OCT) and slit-lamp photographs [17]. The short-term outcomes demonstrated promising reductions in IOP and medication dependency, validating the efficacy and safety of the XEN gel stent in a conjunctiva-sparing approach.

Based on previous research findings, this study extended the follow-up period to 24 months for the same patient cohort to examine the long-term efficacy, safety, and stability of the XEN gel stent. By analyzing the evolution of bleb morphology and clinical outcomes using AS-OCT images and slit-lamp examinations, our goal is to identify reliable predictors of sustained surgical success. This research aims to significantly advance the understanding of MIGS, particularly the ab interno approach with the XEN gel stent, providing crucial insights for optimizing glaucoma management strategies.

2. Materials and Methods

2.1. Study Enrollment

In this retrospective single-center study, the electronic medical records of all patients who underwent XEN gel stent surgery for medically uncontrolled POAG or PXG at the CHA Bundang Medical Center between November 2018 and June 2019 were reviewed and consecutively enrolled. This study was approved by the Institutional Review Board of the CHA Bundang Medical Center and conducted at the CHA Glaucoma Clinic of the CHA Bundang Medical Center in accordance with the tenets of the Declaration of Helsinki. Written informed consent was obtained from all patients without a waiver.

2.2. Surgical Success Definitions

Success was defined as achieving an IOP of less than 14 mmHg and more than 20% reduction in preoperative IOP, with no additional glaucoma surgery or findings of vision-threatening complications. This includes qualified success, with or without any ocular hypotensive medications, and complete success, without any ocular hypotensive medications. Needling was not considered as glaucoma surgery. Hypotony was defined as having an IOP of less than 6 mm Hg at any visit.

2.3. Surgical Procedures

All surgical procedures were performed by a skilled surgeon (S.R.) after obtaining informed consent from all patients, following procedures outlined in previous studies [17]. Briefly, after topical anesthesia, 0.05 mL of 2% lidocaine with epinephrine was injected into the superior subconjunctival space, 6 mm from the XEN tip site. Viscoelastics were injected via a 1 mm side port to maintain the anterior chamber. The XEN injector, through a 1.5 mm corneal incision, placed the XEN implant 2 mm from the limbus at the superonasal angle. Confirmation via surgical gonioscopy was followed by viscoelastic removal, corneal wound sealing with balanced salt solution hydrosealing, and subconjunctival MMC injection (0.05 mL, 0.2–0.4 mg/mL).

2.4. Follow-Up and Outcome Measures

Patients were followed up on postoperative day 1, week 1, month 1, month 3, month 6, month 12, month 18, and month 24. During each visit, IOP measurement, best-corrected visual acuity (BCVA) assessment, slit-lamp examination, corneal endothelial cell count examination, and AS-OCT were performed. The primary outcome evaluated the surgical success rate by assessing the reduction in IOP and the change in the number of medications compared with baseline in the 2-year follow-up after XEN gel stent surgery. Secondary outcome measures included evaluating long-term surgical outcomes at 2 years based on bleb morphology classified early postoperatively by AS-OCT or slit-lamp examination after surgery. The tip location of the XEN stent was categorized into three groups based on its anatomical position: intraconjunctival, when the tip was located beneath the conjunctiva; intratenon, when the tip was positioned along the interface between the conjunctiva and Tenon's capsule; and uviform, when the tip was obscured by multiple protuberances within a poorly hydrated bleb, making precise localization difficult.

2.5. Statistical Analysis

All data were analyzed using SPSS software version 29.0 (IBM Corp., Armonk, NY, USA). Descriptive statistics were used to summarize the baseline characteristics of the study population. Continuous variables were represented as mean ± standard deviation (SD), while categorical variables were represented as frequencies and percentages. All statistical tests were two-tailed, and a p-value < 0.05 was considered statistically significant. The baseline characteristics were compared between the success and failure groups. Independent t-tests were used for continuous variables such as age, axial length, central corneal thickness (CCT), preoperative visual field index (VFI), preoperative IOP, the number of preoperative medications, and postoperative 1 week IOP. For categorical variables such as sex, the presence of POAG, and PXG, Fisher's exact test was employed to assess the association between these variables and surgical outcomes. The Kruskal–Wallis test was conducted to compare the means among three independent groups due to the small sample size in each group. To evaluate the postoperative course of IOP, number of medications, and ECC changes over time, repeated measures ANOVA was employed to compare the mean values at multiple time points (preoperative, 1 month, 6 months, 12 months, 18 months, and 24 months) within each group (complete success and qualified success). A post hoc test was conducted to identify specific time points where significant differences occurred between the groups. For the non-parametric data related to the number of medications, the Wilcoxon signed-rank test was used to calculate statistical significance. For the analysis of success or failure at 2 years based on bleb morphology via AS-OCT imaging and slit-lamp photography, Fisher's exact test was used due to the relatively small sample sizes in some of the bleb morphology categories.

3. Results

3.1. Demographics of Success and Failure Groups

A standard ab interno XEN implantation was performed in 31 eyes of 31 patients who were followed for at least 2 years. According to the definition of success, as described in the Methods section, the demographic features of the groups that achieved complete success versus failure and qualified success versus failure are summarized in Table 1. No statistically significant difference was observed between the complete success and failure groups, as well as the qualified success and failure groups, regarding age, sex, axial length, CCT, preoperative VFI, preoperative IOP, preoperative medications, the concentration of MMC (0.02% or 0.04%) used, and proportion of POAG and PXG.

Table 1. Clinical characteristics of patients treated with XEN gel stent.

	Qualified Success			Complete Success		
	No (n = 15)	Yes (n = 16)	p-Value	No (n = 20)	Yes (n = 11)	p-Value
Age	64.20 ± 15.51	69.13 ± 15.03	0.874	66.40 ± 14.57	67.36 ± 17.04	0.408
Sex (female, %)	8 (57.1%)	6 (42.9%)	1.000	6 (46.2%)	7 (53.8%)	0.449
Axial length (mm)	25.39	24.69	0.260	25.06	24.98	0.820
CCT (um)	513.33	528.44	0.066	519.10	524.	0.322
Preoperative VFI (%)	44.33	55.13	0.329	45.45	58.3	0.291
Preoperative IOP (mmHg)	29.67	29.0	0.905	28.65	30.6	0.576
Preoperative medications (n)	3.13 ± 1.13	3.06 ± 1.24	0.965	2.95 ± 1.23	3.36 ± 1.03	0.576
MMC			0.504			0.273
0.02% MMC	60.0%	43.7%		60.0%	36.4%	
0.04% MMC	40.0%	56.3%		40.0%	63.6%	
POAG (%)	53.3	81.3	0.135	55.0	90.9	0.055
PXG (%)	46.7	18.7	0.135	45.0	9.1	0.055

sCCT, central corneal thickness; VFI, visual field index; IOP, intraocular pressure; MMC, mitomycin C; POAG, primary open-angle glaucoma; PXG, pseudoexfoliative glaucoma. Values are presented as mean ± standard deviation unless otherwise indicated.

3.2. Surgical Success

Based on the tip location on postoperative day 1, the success rates at 2 years postoperatively were assessed. For complete success, the rates were 33.3% for intraconjunctiva, 38.9% for intratenon, and 28.6% for uviform tip locations (Figure 1a). For qualified success, the rates were 50.0% for intraconjunctiva, 50.0% for intratenon, and 57.1% for uviform tip locations (Figure 1b). The Kruskal–Wallis test indicated that the differences in success rates among the intraconjunctiva, intratenon, and uviform groups were not statistically significant for both complete success and qualified success (p = 0.268 and p = 0.637, respectively).

In the complete success group, IOP was significantly lower at 1, 6, 12, 18, and 24 months postoperatively compared with the failure group (Figure 2a). In the qualified success group, IOP remained consistently lower than in the failure group after 6 months postoperatively (Figure 2b). The number of intraocular pressure-lowering medications was not significantly different between the success groups (qualified and complete success) and the two failure groups preoperatively. However, the complete success group required consistently fewer medications than the failure group after 6 months postoperatively (Figure 2c). The qualified success group did not show a statistically significant difference in the number of medications at any time point except at 18 months postoperatively (Figure 2d). The change in endothelial cell count (ECC) showed a significant difference between the complete success and failure groups at 2 years, but no statistically significant differences were observed between the success groups (qualified and complete success) and the two failure groups at other times.

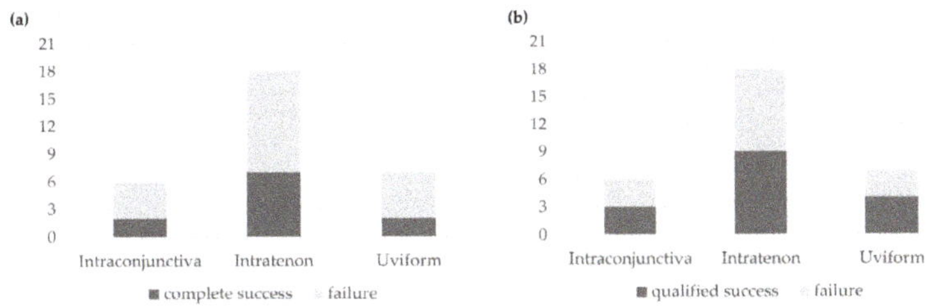

Figure 1. Success or failure at the 2 years of complete success (**a**) and qualified success (**b**) rates by the number of patients in relation to the intraconjunctiva, intratenon, and uviform tip locations based on the tip location on the 1st postoperative day. (**a**) $p = 0.268$, (**b**) $p = 0.637$ (Kruskal–Wallis test).

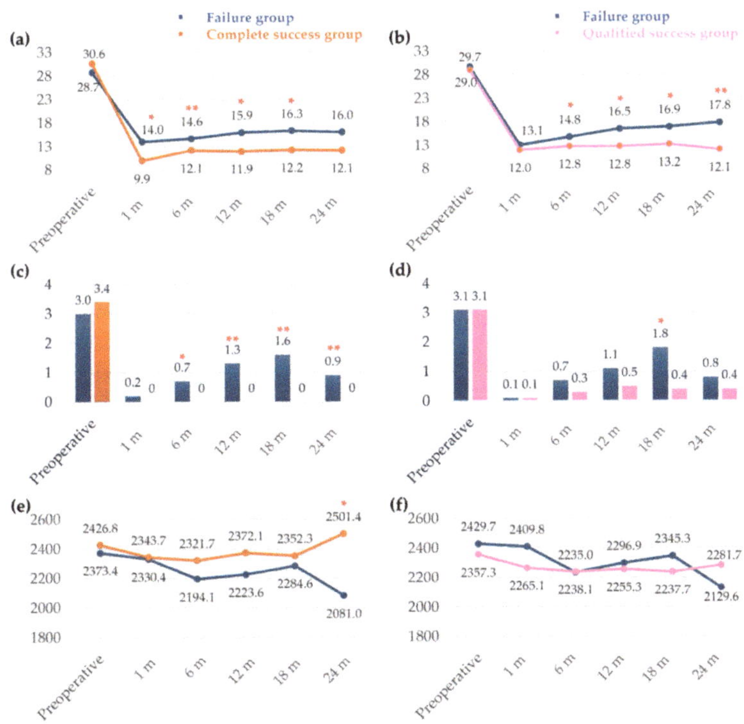

Figure 2. Mean IOP changes (**a**,**b**), number of medications (**c**,**d**), and change in ECC (**e**,**f**) over time in the complete success group (**a**,**c**,**e**) and qualified success group (**b**,**d**,**f**) compared with the failure group preoperatively and at 1 month, 6 months, 12 months, 18 months, and 24 months postoperatively. IOP, intraocular pressure (mmHg); ECC, endothelial cell count (*, $p < 0.05$; **, $p < 0.01$).

Based on the analysis of bleb morphology using AS-OCT at 6 months postoperatively, the surgical success at 2 years postoperatively was evaluated. In the complete success group, the high sparse wall group at 6 months postoperatively had a statistically significantly higher success rate compared with other morphologies ($p = 0.007$) (Figure 3a). In the qualified success group, there was no statistically significant difference in success rate at 2 years based on bleb morphology (Figure 3b). Based on the classification of bleb morphology groups using slit-lamp photography at 6 months postoperatively, the surgical success rate at 2 years was significantly higher in the avascular group than in the vascular group for both complete success ($p = 0.009$) (Figure 3c) and qualified success groups ($p = 0.038$) (Figure 3d).

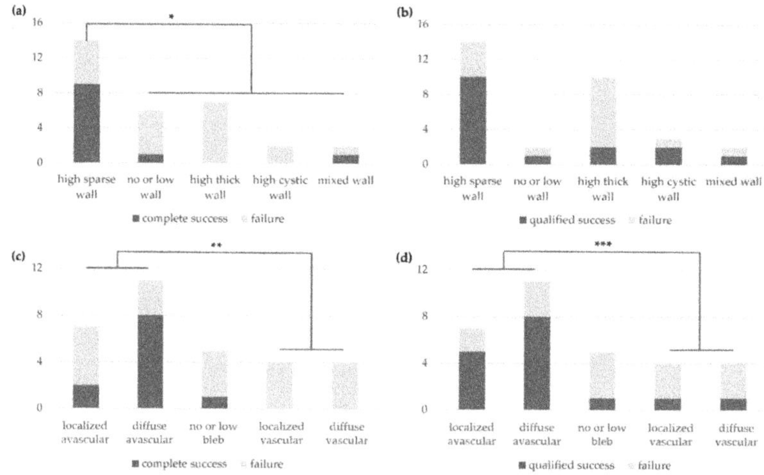

Figure 3. Success or failure at the 2 years of complete success (**a**) or qualified success (**b**) according to bleb morphology via AS-OCT imaging and complete success (**c**) or qualified success (**d**) according to bleb morphology via slit-lamp photography at 6 months postoperatively (*, $p = 0.007$; **, $p = 0.009$; ***, $p = 0.038$).

At 2 years postoperatively, complete success was most observed in the high sparse wall type ($p = 0.038$) as classified by AS-OCT (Figure 4a), while there was no difference in success rates among bleb morphologies for qualified success (Figure 4b). Additionally, based on slit-lamp photography at 2 years postoperatively, the avascular type demonstrated a higher surgical success rate compared with the vascular type ($p = 0.044$) (Figure 4c), with no difference observed based on bleb morphology for qualified success (Figure 4d).

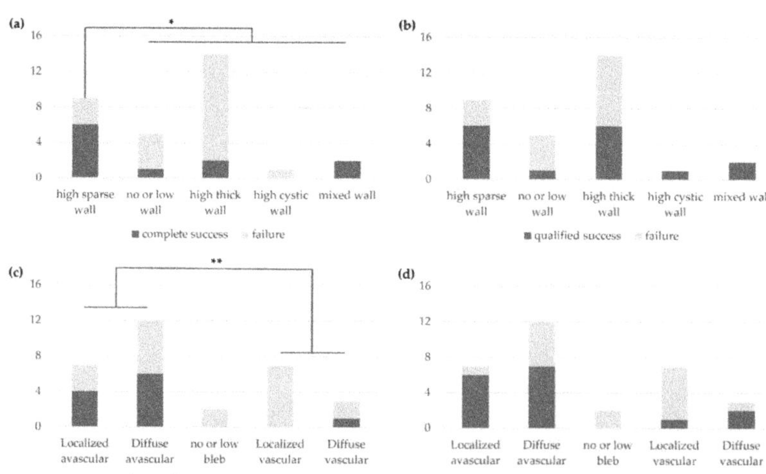

Figure 4. Success or failure at 2 years of complete success (**a**) or qualified success (**b**) according to bleb morphology via AS-OCT imaging and complete success (**c**) or qualified success (**d**) according to bleb morphology via slit-lamp photography at 2 years postoperatively (*, $p = 0.038$; **, $p = 0.044$).

3.3. Postoperative Interventions

Needling was performed in 10 eyes (32.3%) out of 31, and a total of 18 needling procedures were performed. Among the eyes that received needling, the proportion of those requiring one and two procedures was the same (12.9%), while 2 eyes (6.5%) underwent three needling procedures. A secondary surgical procedure was performed in a total of 5 eyes (16.1%), with 3 eyes undergoing trabeculectomy and 3 eyes (9.7%) and 2 eyes (6.5%) undergoing XEN revision (Table 2).

Table 2. Postoperative interventions and secondary surgical procedure.

Interventions	Number of Eyes (%) (n = 31)
Needling	10 (32.3)
1×	4 (12.9)
2×	4 (12.9)
3×	2 (6.5)
Secondary surgical procedure	5 (16.1)
Trabeculectomy	3 (9.7)
XEN revision	2 (6.5)

3.4. Safety

Regarding the safety profile, hypotony was the most common complication. It occurred in 21 eyes (67.7%) on the 1st postoperative day, 7 eyes (22.6%) at 1 week postoperatively, and 1 eye (3.2%) at 1 month postoperatively. There were no cases of hypotony at 6 months, 1 year, or 2 years postoperatively. The incidence of ocular adverse events, excluding hypotony, was observed in 10 eyes (32.3%). Hyphema was the most common, occurring in 4 eyes (12.9%) and resolved spontaneously within 14 days postoperatively. Choroidal detachment occurred in 3 eyes (9.5%). Vitreous hemorrhage and tube bending each occurred in 2 eyes (6.5%), while tube migration occurred in 1 eye (3.2%) (Table 3).

Table 3. Adverse events reported throughout the 2-year follow-up. * Intraocular pressure < 6 mmHg.

Adverse Events	Number of Eyes (%) (n = 31)
Hypotony *	
POD 1d	21 (67.7)
POD 1w	7 (22.6)
POD 1m	1 (3.2)
POD 6m	0 (0.0)
POD 12m	0 (0.0)
POD 24m	0 (0.0)
Hyphema	4 (12.9)
Vitreous hemorrhage	2 (6.5)
Tube bending	2 (6.5)
Tube migration	1 (3.2)
Choroidal detachment	1 (3.2)

4. Discussion

One of the most notable observations in this study is the association between bleb morphology observed through slit-lamp examination and AS-OCT imaging at 6 months postoperatively and surgical success at 2 years. While this finding suggests a potential predictive value, further validation in larger prospective studies is warranted. Notably, patients with high sparse wall or avascular bleb morphology at 6 months tended to maintain higher surgical success rates at 2 years. Using AS-OCT, known for its high reliability in evaluating intraocular structures and providing accurate repeated measurements [19], Lenzhofer et al. reported that the XEN gel stent resulted in a higher proportion of uniform blebs (48%) compared with trabeculectomy, with significantly greater bleb height and internal cavity presence at 6 months ($p = 0.031$, $p < 0.001$) and 1 year ($p = 0.039$, $p = 0.001$), and lower postoperative IOP in the internal cavity group at both time points ($p = 0.024$, $p = 0.040$) [20]. These findings align with Seoyoung Wy's observations that blebs with an internal cavity, or diffuse subconjunctival cysts, had lower postoperative IOP and better regulated aqueous humor outflow due to the cavity height [18]. These bleb morphologies suggest that AS-OCT imaging can serve as an important indicator for predicting long-term surgical success, along with more stable IOP reduction. Our previous study on the 6-month follow-up data revealed that postoperative IOP at 1 week and female gender were significantly associated with higher success rates [17]. This suggested that early postoperative IOP and gender could be potential predictors of surgical success in the short term. However, in the current study's long-term follow-up at 2 years, we observed that neither postoperative IOP at 1 week nor gender had a significant impact on the success rates. This discrepancy between the short-term and long-term predictors highlights the dynamic nature of surgical outcomes and suggests that early indicators might not necessarily translate into long-term success. This discrepancy may be due to the progressive remodeling of the bleb and surrounding tissues over time, which cannot be fully predicted by early IOP alone. Initial IOP reduction may reflect immediate surgical success but not necessarily indicate sustained outflow function. These findings underscore the importance of mid-term assessments, such as AS-OCT imaging at 6 months, as more reliable indicators of long-term outcomes, and highlight the need for continued postoperative monitoring beyond the early postoperative period. They also emphasize the importance of evaluating multiple factors over an extended period to accurately predict surgical outcomes. Additionally, it is important to note that bleb morphology can change over time with follow-up, potentially affecting long-term success rates. This shift in predictive factors from short-term to long-term outcomes is an intriguing aspect of our study, shedding light on the complex and evolving nature of bleb morphology and its influence on surgical success.

In a large-scale retrospective multicenter observational study involving 646 eyes, the complete success ($6 \leq \text{IOP} \leq 18$ mmHg, no medication) and qualified success ($6 \leq \text{IOP} \leq 18$ mmHg, with medication) rates at 2 years postoperatively were 26% and 48%, respectively [21]. Reitsamer et al. reported a clinical success rate (≥20% IOP reduction, same or fewer medications without secondary surgical intervention) of 67.6% at 12 months and 65.8% at 24 months [22]. Grover et al. evaluated the 12-month outcomes of standalone XEN implantation in 65 patients with refractory glaucoma, finding that 75.4% of eyes achieved more than a 20% reduction in IOP while using a similar or fewer number of medications [23]. In a cohort of 129 eyes, 54.2% achieved more than a 20% reduction in IOP and maintained an IOP of less than 18 mmHg for 24 months following standalone XEN surgery [24]. Using the 16 mmHg threshold, 51.4% (POAG) versus 57.1% (PXG) eyes achieved complete success ($p = 0.70$) at 2 years [25]. This shows that the notable advantage of the PXG group over the POAG cohort during the first 12 months is no longer statistically significant, as observed by the same authors. We defined the success criterion for IOP as being less than 14 mmHg, which is even more strict than in other study designs. In our study, the complete success rate at 2 years was 35.5% (11/31), and the qualified success rate was 51.6% (16/31), which seems to have lower success rates compared with other studies. Rauchegger et al. reported that complete surgical success was achieved in 39% of patients at 12 months and 34% at 24 months, with qualified success in 29% at 12 months and 27% at 24 months, while 13 eyes (16%) were classified as complete surgical failure [9]. The minimal change in success rates from 12 months to 24 months postoperatively highlights the long-term stability of the XEN gel stent. Thus, the XEN gel stent can be considered a safe and effective long-term treatment option for glaucoma.

In our study, needling was performed in 10 out of 31 eyes (32.3%), with a total of 18 needling procedures conducted. Patrica et al. reported a needling rate of 19% in 94 patients who underwent a standardized needling technique over 1 year [26], while Grover et al. evaluated 65 patients with refractory glaucoma who received XEN45 with mitomycin C 0.2 mg/mL and disclosed needling rates of 32% [23]. A study performed in Portugal involving 15 eyes undergoing XEN with MMC 0.2 mg/mL had a 33% needling rate 3 months after surgery [26]. A recent study published by Midha et al. reported an overall needling rate of 45% over 24 months [27]. Reitsamer et al. and Gabbay et al. reported needling rates of 41.1% and 37.7%, respectively, after 2 years of follow-up [22,28], while Tan et al. reported a needling rate of 51.3% after 1 year [10]. High needling rate could be attributed to our proactive approach to managing bleb function early in the postoperative period. Ensuring optimal bleb function is crucial in the early months following surgery to prevent fibrosis and scarring, which can lead to surgical failure.

The use of intraoperative MMC during XEN implant surgery has become standard practice [1,2,5,7,9,17,18,20–23,26]. Natalia et al. investigated the efficacy and safety of two MMC doses (0.01% vs. 0.02%) in eyes undergoing XEN45 implantation, either alone or with phacoemulsification, and found no significant differences in IOP reduction, hypotensive medication use, or adverse events between the doses [29]. The results suggest that lower doses might be feasible, although MMC 0.01% did not reduce adverse events [29]. A study on standalone XEN45 gel stent implantation reported a therapeutic success rate of 39% without MMC and 55% with MMC at 1 year, while the failure rates were 61% without MMC and 45% with MMC, indicating that MMC use appeared to increase the therapeutic success rate, though it did not reach statistical significance [30].

Regarding XEN45, the concentration of MMC could potentially affect clinical outcomes. Some research suggests that the success rate might be linked to the MMC dose, although other studies have found no correlation between MMC dosage and surgical results [31]. In our study, we used MMC at concentrations of 0.02% and 0.04%, but no significant difference in success rates was observed between these concentrations, suggesting that the concentration of MMC may not be a critical factor in determining the success of the procedure. Additionally, there is a report of severe complication where MMC toxicity led to significant eye pain and a large avascular bleb [32].

Currently, there is no definitive evidence to support the use of a particular MMC concentration. Therefore, it might be advisable to use the lowest effective dose of MMC as judged by the surgeon for the specific patient. Nonetheless, further research is needed to provide clearer guidance on this matter. In particular, identifying the optimal and least hazardous concentration of MMC should be a key focus of future investigations.

XEN has emerged as a safe and less invasive method for lowering IOP in glaucoma patients, but it is still not free from complications. Hypotony (IOP < 6 mmHg) is the most common complication, occurring in approximately 4.0–27.0% of cases [21,22,33,34]. Nicolaou et al. reported that numerical hypotony (IOP ≤ 6 mmHg) occurred at any point in 75 of 186 cases (40%), and no significant visual acuity deficit remained 4 weeks after surgery [12]. In our study, we observed a hypotony rate of 67.6% (10 eyes) on the 1st postoperative day. The higher rate of hypotony in our study compared with that in other studies may be attributed to the fact that we included measurements taken on the 1st postoperative day, whereas most other studies measured the incidence at 1 month or 6 months postoperatively. However, the hypotony rate in our study decreased to 3.2%

(1 eye) by the 1st month postoperatively and was not observed again. Notably, all cases of hypotony resolved within 2 to 3 months without long-term adverse effects, highlighting the transient nature of this complication when managed properly.

Secondary glaucoma surgeries following XEN implantation have been reported to occur in 10.4–41.5% of cases [9,21,22,34–36]. Our study observed that secondary surgical procedures were necessary in 5 out of 31 eyes (16.1%) within the 1st 2 years, with 3 eyes undergoing trabeculectomy and 2 eyes undergoing XEN revision. This finding aligns with that of Rauchegger et al., who reported a 16% (n = 13) rate of secondary interventions, including trabeculectomy (11%, n = 9) and repeat XEN implantation (5%, n = 4) [9]. This indicates that, despite the initial success of the XEN gel stent, some patients still required additional surgical intervention to maintain adequate IOP control regarding stent occlusion or bleb fibrosis.

This study, despite its small sample size, followed up all 31 patients from a previously reported study for a period of 2 years after surgery, providing long-term outcome data. This comprehensive follow-up underscores that our findings reflect real-world data. Additionally, this study focused on naïve patients with no prior glaucoma surgery, which limits direct comparisons with the outcomes of XEN implantation in patients with secondary glaucoma. Lastly, the criteria for needling were based on AS-OCT morphology and the absence of tube occlusion, with YAG laser being used for cases of tube occlusion. Therefore, the needling procedures and their timing were not standardized and were left to the discretion of the experienced surgeon (S.R.). This variability could influence the outcomes and makes it challenging to draw definitive conclusions about the efficacy of needling in managing bleb function. Standardized protocols for needling interventions should be established and evaluated in future studies to determine the optimal timing and technique for improving surgical outcomes. In addition, comparative studies with other MIGS, such as iStent, Hydrus, or Preserflo, would provide further insights on the relative efficacy and safety of the XEN gel stent and help clarify its clinical role among current surgical options. Furthermore, long-term follow-up beyond 2 years is warranted to evaluate the sustained effectiveness and safety of the XEN gel stent and to determine whether the favorable outcomes observed in this study are maintained over time.

5. Conclusions

In conclusion, the ab interno XEN gel stent showed favorable 2-year outcomes in patients with POAG and PXG. High sparse wall and avascular bleb types at 6 months were associated with greater long-term success, highlighting the prognostic value of mid-term AS-OCT imaging. These findings support the importance of structured postoperative monitoring in sustaining surgical efficacy.

Author Contributions: Study concept and design, D.K. and S.R.; collection and management of data, D.K. and S.R.; analysis and interpretation of data, D.K., M.K., M.L. and S.R.; statistical analysis, D.K.; writing and review of the manuscript, D.K. and S.R. All authors have read and agreed to the published version of the manuscript.

Funding: This research received no external funding.

Institutional Review Board Statement: The study and the data collection protocol were approved by the Institutional Review Board of the CHA Bundang Medical Center, Seongnam, South Korea (IRB File No. CHAMC 2024-07-046, Approved on 14 August in 2024). This study adhered to the tenets of the Declaration of Helsinki.

Informed Consent Statement: Informed consent was obtained from all subjects involved in this study.

Data Availability Statement: The datasets analyzed during the current study are available from the corresponding author on reasonable requests.

Conflicts of Interest: The authors declare no conflicts of interest.

References

1. Lewis, R.A. Ab interno approach to the subconjunctival space using a collagen glaucoma stent. *J. Cataract. Refract. Surg.* **2014**, *40*, 1301–1306. [CrossRef] [PubMed]
2. Gedde, S.J.; Vinod, K.; Prum, B.E., Jr.; Primary Tube Versus Trabeculectomy Study Group. Results from the Primary Tube Versus Trabeculectomy Study and translation to clinical practice. *Curr. Opin. Ophthalmol.* **2023**, *34*, 129–137. [CrossRef] [PubMed]
3. Yang, S.A.; Mitchell, W.; Hall, N.; Elze, T.; Lorch, A.C.; Miller, J.W.; Zebardast, N.; IRIS® Registry Data Analytics Consortium. Trends and Usage Patterns of Minimally Invasive Glaucoma Surgery in the United States: IRIS® Registry Analysis 2013–2018. *Ophthalmol. Glaucoma* **2021**, *4*, 558–568. [CrossRef]
4. Sheybani, A. The Future of Glaucoma Surgery. *J. Ophthalmic. Vis. Res.* **2015**, *10*, 340–341. [CrossRef] [PubMed]
5. Cappelli, F.; Cutolo, C.A.; Olivari, S.; Testa, V.; Sindaco, D.; Pizzorno, C.; Ciccione, S.; Traaverso, C.E.; Iester, M. Trabeculectomy versus Xen gel implant for the treatment of open-angle glaucoma: A 3-year retrospective analysis. *BMJ Open Ophthalmol.* **2022**, *7*, e000830. [CrossRef]
6. Chen, X.Z.; Liang, Z.Q.; Yang, K.Y.; Lv, K.; Ma, Y.; Li, M.Y.; Wu, H.J. The Outcomes of XEN Gel Stent Implantation: A Systematic Review and Meta-Analysis. *Front. Med.* **2022**, *9*, 804847. [CrossRef] [PubMed]
7. Gillmann, K.; Bravetti, G.E.; Rao, H.L.; Mermoud, A.; Mansouri, K. Impact of Phacoemulsification Combined with XEN Gel Stent Implantation on Corneal Endothelial Cell Density: 2-Year Results. *J. Glaucoma* **2020**, *29*, 155–160. [CrossRef]
8. Oddone, F.; Roberti, G.; Posarelli, C.; Agnifili, L.; Mastropasqua, L.; Carnevale, C.; Micelli Ferrari, T.; Pace, V.; Sacchi, M.; Cremonesi, E.; et al. Endothelial Cell Density After XEN Implant Surgery: Short-term Data from the Italian XEN Glaucoma Treatment Registry (XEN-GTR). *J. Glaucoma* **2021**, *30*, 559–565. [CrossRef]
9. Rauchegger, T.; Angermann, R.; Willeit, P.; Schmid, E.; Teuchner, B. Two-year outcomes of minimally invasive XEN Gel Stent implantation in primary open-angle and pseudoexfoliation glaucoma. *Acta Ophthalmol.* **2021**, *99*, 369–375. [CrossRef]
10. Tan, S.Z.; Walkden, A.; Au, L. One-year result of XEN45 implant for glaucoma: Efficacy, safety, and postoperative management. *Eye* **2018**, *32*, 324–332. [CrossRef]
11. Torbey, T.; Mansouri, K.; Gillmann, K.; Mermoud, A.; Achache, A.R. XEN45 gel stent implantation in open-angle glaucoma: 5-year results of a prospective study. *J. Glaucoma* **2023**, *32*, 909–917. [CrossRef] [PubMed]
12. Nicolaou, S.; Khatib, T.Z.; Lin, Z.; Sheth, T.; Ogbonna, G.; Hamidovic, L.; Zaheer, A.; Dimitriou, C. A retrospective review of XEN implant surgery: Efficacy, safety and the effect of combined cataract surgery. *Int. Ophthalmol.* **2022**, *42*, 881–889. [CrossRef]
13. Hohberger, B.; Welge-LuBen, U.C.; Lammer, R. MIGS: Therapeutic success of combined Xen Gel Stent implantation with cataract surgery. *Graefes Arch. Clin. Exp. Ophthalmol.* **2018**, *256*, 621–625. [CrossRef] [PubMed]
14. Karimi, A.; Lindfield, D.; Turnbull, A.; Dimitriou, C.; Bhatia, B.; Radwan, M.; Gouws, P.; Hanifudin, A.; Amerasinghe, N.; Jocob, A. A multi-centre interventional case series of 259 ab-interno Xen gel implants for glaucoma, with and without combined cataract surgery. *Eye* **2019**, *33*, 469–477. [CrossRef]
15. Olgun, A.; Duzgun, E.; Yildiz, A.M.; Atmaca, F.; Yildiz, A.A.; Sendul, S.Y. XEN Gel Stent versus trabeculectomy: Short-term effects on corneal endothelial cells. *Eur. J. Ophthalmol.* **2021**, *31*, 346–353. [CrossRef] [PubMed]
16. Marcos-Parra, M.T.; Mendoza-Moreira, A.L.; Moreno-Castro, L.; Mateos-Marcos, C.; Salinas Lopez, J.A.; Figuerola-Garcia, M.B.; Gonzalez-Alonso, A.; Perez-Santonja, J.J. 3-Year outcomes of XEN implant compared with trabeculectomy, with or without phacoemulsification for open-angle glaucoma. *J. Glaucoma* **2022**, *31*, 826–833. [CrossRef]
17. Kim, Y.; Lim, S.H.; Rho, S. Bleb Analysis Using Anterior Segment Optical Coherence Tomography and Surgical Predictors of XEN Gel Stent. *Transl. Vis. Sci. Technol.* **2022**, *11*, 26. [CrossRef]
18. Wy, S.; Shin, Y.I.; Kim, Y.K.; Jeoung, J.W.; Park, K.H. Bleb Morphology on Anterior-Segment Optical Coherence Tomography after XEN Gel Stent Implantation. *J. Clin. Med.* **2023**, *12*, 6740. [CrossRef]
19. Yuan, L.; Rana, H.S.; Lee, I.; Lai, G.; Raiciulescu, S.; Kim, W. Short-Term Outcomes of Xen-45 Gel Stent Ab Interno Versus Ab Externo Transconjunctival Approaches. *J. Glaucoma* **2023**, *32*, e71–e79. [CrossRef]
20. Lenzhofer, M.; Strohmaier, C.; Hohensinn, M.; Hitzl, W.; Sperl, P.; Gerner, M.; Steiner, V.; Moussa, S.; Krall, E.; Reitsamer, H.A. Longitudinal bleb morphology in anterior segment OCT after minimally invasive transscleral ab interno Glaucoma Gel Microstent implantation. *Acta Ophthalmol.* **2019**, *97*, e231–e237. [CrossRef]
21. Arnould, L.; Balsat, E.; Hashimoto, Y.; White, A.; Kong, G.; Dunn, H.; Fan, L.; Gabrielle, P.H.; Bron, A.M.; Creuzot-Garcher, C.P.; et al. Two-year outcomes of Xen 45 gel stent implantation in patients with open-angle glaucoma: Real-world data from the Fight Glaucoma Blindness registry. *Br. J. Ophthalmol.* **2024**, *108*, 1672–1678. [CrossRef]

22. Reitsamer, H.; Sng, C.; Vera, V.; Lenzhofer, M.; Barton, K.; Stalmans, I.; Apex Study Group. Two-year results of a multicenter study of the ab interno gelatin implant in medically uncontrolled primary open-angle glaucoma. *Graefes Arch. Clin. Exp. Ophthalmol.* **2019**, *257*, 983–996. [CrossRef]
23. Grover, D.S.; Flynn, W.J.; Bashford, K.P.; Lewis, R.A.; Duh, Y.J.; Nangia, R.S.; Niksch, B. Performance and Safety of a New Ab Interno Gelatin Stent in Refractory Glaucoma at 12 Months. *Am. J. Ophthalmol.* **2017**, *183*, 25–36. [CrossRef]
24. Mansouri, K.; Bravetti, G.E.; Gillmann, K.; Rao, H.L.; Ch'ng, T.W.; Mermoud, A. Two-Year Outcomes of XEN Gel Stent Surgery in Patients with Open-Angle Glaucoma. *Ophthalmol. Glaucoma* **2019**, *2*, 309–318. [CrossRef] [PubMed]
25. Gillmann, K.; Bravetti, G.E.; Mermoud, A.; Rao, H.L.; Mansouri, K. XEN Gel Stent in Pseudoexfoliative Glaucoma: 2-Year Results of a Prospective Evaluation. *J. Glaucoma* **2019**, *28*, 676–684. [CrossRef] [PubMed]
26. Jose, P.; Teixeira, F.J.; Barao, R.C.; Sens, P.; Abegao Pinto, L. Needling after XEN gel implant: What's the efficacy? A 1-year analysis. *Eur. J. Ophthalmol.* **2021**, *31*, 3087–3092. [CrossRef] [PubMed]
27. Midha, N.; Gillmann, K.; Chaudhary, A.; Mermoud, A.; Mansouri, K. Efficacy of Needling Revision After XEN Gel Stent Implantation: A Prospective Study. *J. Glaucoma* **2020**, *29*, 11–14. [CrossRef]
28. Gabbay, I.E.; Allen, F.; Morley, C.; Pearsall, T.; Bowes, O.M.; Ruben, S. Efficacy and safety data for the XEN45 implant at 2 years: A retrospective analysis. *Br. J. Ophthalmol.* **2020**, *104*, 1125–1130. [CrossRef]
29. Monja-Alarcon, N.; Perucho-Martinez, S.; Buenasmananas-Maeso, M.; Toledano-Fernandez, N. Does mitomycin-C concentration have any influence on XEN45 gel stent outcomes in a real-world setting? *Graefes Arch. Clin. Exp. Ophthalmol.* **2022**, *260*, 2649–2661. [CrossRef]
30. Denkel, L.; Hohberger, B.; Lammer, R. Influence of Mitomycin C on the Therapeutic Success of Stand-Alone Xen45 Gel Stents and Its Combination with Cataract Surgery in Open-Angle Glaucoma Patients. *Klin. Monbl. Augenheilkd.* **2021**, *238*, 861–867. [CrossRef]
31. Bell, K.; de Padua Soares Bezerra, B.; Mofokeng, M.; Montesano, G.; Nongpiur, M.E.; Marti, M.V.; Lawlor, M. Learning from the past: Mitomycin C use in trabeculectomy and its application in bleb-forming minimally invasive glaucoma surgery. *Surv. Ophthalmol.* **2021**, *66*, 109–123. [CrossRef] [PubMed]
32. Baeg, J.Y.; Choi, H.S.; Lee, S.H. A case of mitomycin C toxicity after XEN gel stent implantation with the XEN air technique in a glaucoma patient. *BMC Ophthalmol.* **2023**, *23*, 407. [CrossRef] [PubMed]
33. Hengerer, F.H.; Kohnen, T.; Mueller, M.; Conrad-Hengerer, I. Ab Interno Gel Implant for the Treatment of Glaucoma Patients with or Without Prior Glaucoma Surgery: 1-Year Results. *J. Glaucoma* **2017**, *26*, 1130–1136. [CrossRef]
34. Bravetti, G.E.; Mansouri, K.; Gillmann, K.; Rao, H.L.; Mermoud, A. XEN-augmented Baerveldt drainage device implantation in refractory glaucoma: 1-year outcomes. *Graefes Arch. Clin. Exp. Ophthalmol.* **2020**, *258*, 1787–1794. [CrossRef] [PubMed]
35. Marcos-Parra, M.T.; Salinas-Lopez, J.A.; Mateos-Marcos, C.; Moreno-Castro, L.; Mendoza-Moreira, A.L.; Perez-Santonja, J.J. Long-Term Effectiveness of XEN 45 Gel-Stent in Open-Angle Glaucoma Patients. *Clin. Ophthalmol.* **2023**, *17*, 1223–1232. [CrossRef]
36. Papazoglou, A.; Hohn, R.; Schawkat, M.; Tappeiner, C.; Iliev, M.; Gugleta, K.; Saletta, G.; Wiencierz, A.; Wagels, B.; Todorova, M.G.; et al. Swiss Multicenter Ab Interno XEN45 Gel Stent Study: 2-Year Real-World Data. *Ophthalmol. Ther.* **2024**, *13*, 1513–1525. [CrossRef]

Journal of
Clinical Medicine

MDPI

Article

Comparison of Intraocular Pressure Measurements with Goldmann Applanation Tonometry, iCare, and Tono-Pen in Young Children with Anterior Segment Abnormalities Under General Anesthesia

Matias K. Studer [1], Milko Iliev [1], Christoph Tappeiner [2,3,4], Beatrice E. Frueh [1] and Stephan A. Fraenkl [1,*]

1 Department of Ophthalmology, Inselspital, Bern University Hospital, University of Bern, 3010 Bern, Switzerland; matias.klaus.studer@gmail.com (M.K.S.); miliev44@yahoo.de (M.I.); beatrice.frueh@insel.ch (B.E.F.)
2 Department of Ophthalmology, Pallas Kliniken, 4600 Olten, Switzerland; christoph.tappeiner@pallas-kliniken.ch
3 Department of Ophthalmology, University Hospital Essen, University Duisburg-Essen, 45147 Essen, Germany
4 Medical Faculty, University of Bern, 3008 Bern, Switzerland
* Correspondence: stephan.fraenkl@insel.ch

Abstract: Background: In young patients with suspected elevated intraocular pressure (IOP), examinations under general anesthesia remain the gold standard. This study aimed to compare the reliability of Goldmann applanation tonometry (Perkins), iCare rebound tonometry, and the Tono-Pen in young children under general anesthesia in a clinical setting. **Methods**: This retrospective study included patients under six years of age requiring an ophthalmic examination under general anesthesia. IOP measurements were performed using all three devices, and central corneal thickness (CCT) was recorded for each patient. **Results**: A total of 38 eyes of 19 children (mean age, 1.8 ± 2.1 years) were included. IOP values of all three devices ranged from 5 to 43 mmHg, with a mean CCT of 645.6 ± 135 µm. The Tono-Pen recorded significantly higher IOP values than the Perkins tonometer (15.2 ± 5.5 mmHg vs. 11.1 ± 4.8 mmHg; $p = 0.002$), while no significant differences were observed between Perkins and iCare. CCT was significantly correlated with iCare (r = 0.344, $p = 0.032$) and the Tono-Pen (r = 0.519, $p = 0.001$) but not with Perkins (r = 0.247, $p = 0.129$). Bland–Altman analysis showed a significant slope for inter-device differences, but when excluding IOP values >25 mmHg, the slope was no longer significant. **Conclusions**: Among the devices tested, the Perkins tonometer was the least affected by other parameters such as CCT and IOP values in young patients under general anesthesia, particularly when IOP exceeded 25 mmHg or corneal thickness was increased. In patients with normal corneas and IOP below 25 mmHg, iCare provided comparable accuracy to Perkins, while the Tono-Pen consistently overestimated IOP compared to both devices.

Keywords: intraocular pressure; childhood glaucoma; rebound tonometer

1. Introduction

The accurate measurement of intraocular pressure (IOP) is essential for the diagnosis and management of glaucoma and other ocular conditions [1,2]. Goldmann applanation tonometry (GAT) is widely regarded as the gold standard for IOP measurement in adults due to its high accuracy and reliability [1]. However, IOP measurement in children presents unique challenges, particularly in cases where patient cooperation is limited. Young children, especially those with congenital or developmental eye conditions, often require general anesthesia for precise IOP assessment, making it necessary to use handheld tonometers that can function effectively in this setting [3]. Congenital glaucoma, a rare but serious disease with an incidence of 1 per 10,000 to 20,000 live births, is one of the key conditions that necessitates IOP measurement in young children [4]. Left undiagnosed or untreated, congenital glaucoma can lead to irreversible visual impairment due to optic nerve damage caused by sustained elevated IOP [5]. Monitoring IOP in children with this condition is crucial for timely intervention, including surgical procedures such as trabeculotomy or goniotomy. In cases of anterior segment abnormalities or post-surgical follow-up, repeated IOP assessments under general anesthesia may be required [6]. Traditionally, GAT remains the gold standard for IOP measurement, but it has practical limitations in pediatric patients [7]. Since it requires a slit lamp setup and patient cooperation, its use in young children is often impractical. Therefore, the portable version of GAT, the Perkins tonometer, has been developed and has been used as a gold standard device to measure IOP in lying patients for many years [8]. It has been shown that GAT and Perkins have a very good accordance [3]. But Perkins needs a skilled examiner and is sometime difficult to perform in irregular corneas [9]. As a result, handheld tonometers such as the Tono-Pen and iCare PRO have been developed to facilitate IOP measurement in children, including those under general anesthesia [10]. Such measurements are feasible even in very young infants [11]. These devices offer portability, ease of use, and the ability to obtain measurements in supine or non-cooperative patients, making them valuable alternatives to GAT in pediatric settings.

The Tono-Pen (Tono-Pen® XL, Reichert Technologies, Depew, NY, USA) was introduced in 1987 and has been widely used for pediatric IOP assessment. This device operates on strain gauge technology, where a microsensor detects changes in corneal resistance during applanation [12]. The Tono-Pen is particularly useful for bedridden patients and those under general anesthesia, as it allows for easy one-handed operation while the patient remains in a supine position. Despite its advantages, concerns have been raised about its accuracy in comparison to GAT, with some studies indicating a tendency for the Tono-Pen to slightly overestimate or underestimate IOP depending on corneal properties [13,14].

More recently, rebound tonometry has gained popularity with the introduction of the iCare PRO and other, similar devices. Unlike applanation-based methods, rebound tonometry measures IOP by analyzing the deceleration of a small probe that makes brief contact with the cornea. This method eliminates the need for topical anesthesia [15] and is well-tolerated by children. The iCare PRO and iCare ic200 models are specifically designed for use in supine patients, making them suitable for IOP measurement under general anesthesia. The inbuilt sensor records the movement of a propelled probe and calculates the IOP by the deceleration of the probe after contact with the cornea [10,16]. It is the iCare PRO that is used most frequently in published studies and that demonstrates good concordance with GAT in healthy individuals and in patients with glaucomatous disease [17,18]. Studies have shown that the iCare PRO demonstrates good agreement with GAT in both healthy individuals and glaucoma patients, although differences in corneal biomechanics can affect the readings [19]. A key challenge in device comparisons for pediatric IOP measurement is the influence of the biomechanical properties of the cornea, especially in young children with congenital glaucoma or anterior segment anomalies [20]. In addition to corneal biomechanics, central corneal thickness (CCT) and other factors have been shown to affect IOP readings obtained with different tonometers [19]. Perkins, the Tono-Pen, and iCare all measure IOP differently, and their readings can vary depending on corneal rigidity and thickness [13]. For instance, the Tono-Pen and iCare seem to be more influenced by corneal biomechanics compared to Perkins, which can lead to slight variations in measurements [17].

The purpose of this study is to compare three clinically used devices—Perkins, the Tono-Pen, and the iCare PRO—for measuring IOP in young children under general anesthesia in a routine clinical setting, to assess the agreement between these tonometers and to identify potential systematic differences. This will help ophthalmologists make informed decisions when selecting a tonometer for use in children, particularly those undergoing surgery or requiring frequent IOP monitoring under anesthesia.

2. Materials and Methods

2.1. Study Population

In this retrospective study, data were collected from pediatric patients that underwent intraocular pressure measurements under general anesthesia at the Department of Ophthalmology, Bern University Hospital, Bern, Switzerland. The inclusion criteria were age $\leq$6 years, the indication for ophthalmological examination and IOP measurement under general anesthesia, and clear corneas without scars or evident leucoma. Haab's Striae were not an exclusion criterion. The decision to perform general anesthesia was made by the pediatric ophthalmologist based on clinical necessity—for example, to obtain accurate refraction or reliable IOP measurements in non-cooperative children, or when other diagnostic procedures could not be performed adequately in an awake state. Patients underwent general anesthesia with sevoflurane. Induction of anesthesia was carried out under propofol with sevoflurane 8% in 100% oxygen carrier gas, with maintenance under spontaneous ventilation. Airway maintenance devices were inserted. Afterwards, a drop of oxybuprocaine 0.4% was applied, and IOP measurements were performed as soon as the anesthesia was effective. IOP measurements were initiated within the first minute after topical anesthesia became effective and were completed within five minutes. All IOP measurements were consistently performed by the same examiner.

2.2. Devices and Measurement Methods

The first device used was the iCARE PRO (iCare Finland Oy, Vantaa, Finland). Six consecutive measurements were taken in the right eye. In the case of an acceptable reading (deviation within normal limits as indicated by the device), the same procedure was performed in the left eye. In the case of a larger deviation (deviation outside normal limits as indicated by the device (<15% deviation)) in readings, six new measurements were taken until an acceptable reading was obtained.

The second device used was the Tono-Pen (Reichert Technologies, Depew, NY, USA). First, it had to be calibrated. Four consecutive measurements were taken in the right eye. In the case of a good reliability (deviation < 5%), the same procedure was performed in the left eye. In the case of a high deviation in the readings, the measurement was repeated until a good reliability was obtained.

The third device used was the Perkins tonometer (Haag Streit, Köniz, Switzerland). Fluorescein (BioGlo Fluorescein Sodium strips, HUB Pharmaceuticals, Rancho Cucamonga, Canada) was applied on the tear film and IOP measurement was performed first on the right, and then on the left eye (corresponding to a Goldmann applanation tonometry reading). Care was taken on the proper lubrication of the eyes.

The reason for this sequential testing was to minimize the trauma to the corneal epithelium (for example, after the application of fluorescein and (repeated) applanation with the Perkins tonometer) and its influence on the following exams. The probe of the iCare Pro instrument is the smallest of all three devices, and the physical stress to the cornea is the lowest.

After the IOP readings, central corneal thickness (CCT), corneal diameter, and axial length were measured with an Ultrasonic B scanner UD-8000 (TOMEY, Nagoya, Japan), objective refraction was obtained (Heine Beta 200 Skiaskop, HEINE Optotechnik GmbH, Herrsching, Germany) and gonioscopy and handheld slit-lamp examination (Kowa SL-17, portable slit lamp, Torrance, CA, USA) were performed.

2.3. Statistical Analysis

The comparison of IOP measurements with the three devices was analyzed using the Kruskal–Wallis test followed by the Dunn's post hoc test. A Williams-T-Test was performed to analyze dependent correlations between devices and pachymetry. The Bland–Altmann test was performed to visualize the dependence of two methods and the dependence of readings from pachymetry. This analysis was made for all existing IOP measurements.

In a second step, the analysis was performed a second time by excluding measurements above 25 mmHg in order to evaluate the effect of high IOP readings on the accuracy of the methods. Lines indicate the mean of the differences and +/− two standard deviations (lower, upper limits of agreement). A critical difference indicates two standard deviations. Regression results were reported as slopes with 95% confidence intervals and *p*-values. Slopes were calculated using a linear mixed-effects model. Data analysis was performed using GraphPad Prism Software (version 9.5.1) and the statistical software R (version 3.5.0).

This study was approved by the ethical committee of Bern, Switzerland (BASEC No. 2020-00635) and written informed consent was obtained from all children's parents.

3. Results

A total of 19 children (38 eyes) were included in this study (female n = 11, 58%). Patients were between one month and six years old (mean age 1.8 ± 2.1 years). A total of 18 eyes were aphakic, 10 eyes had a congenital cataract, 7 eyes had congenital glaucoma (1 of them was also aphakic), 3 had a nystagmus and/or hyperopia, and 2 fellow eyes were normal (Table 1). IOP ranged between 5 mmHg and 43 mmHg (iCare: 6–43 mmHg; Tono-Pen: 5–37 mmHg; Perkins: 5–34 mmHg).

Pachymetry was 646 µm ± 135. The corneal diameter measured 10.6 ± 1.4 mm horizontally and 10.1 ± 1.5 mm vertically. Comparing the three devices, the only statistically significant difference between groups was the Tono-Pen compared with the Perkins tonometer, i.e., the Tono-Pen results were higher than the Perkins results (15.2 ± 5.5 mmHg vs. 11.1 ± 4.8 mmHg; $p = 0.02$). The iCare values were slightly higher than those measured with Perkins as well, but this finding was not statistically significant (11.6 mmHg ± 4.4 vs. 11.1 ± 4.8 mmHg; $p > 0.05$).

The best correspondence was between iCare and Perkins. As the measures strongly deviated from normal distributions as evaluated in Q-Q plots, Spearman correlations were calculated. Pachymetric measures were significantly correlated with iCare ($r = 0.344$, $p = 0.032$) and the Tono-Pen ($r = 0.519$, $p = 0.001$) but not Perkins ($r = 0.247$, $p = 0.129$).

There was a significant correlation between the difference between Perkins and the Tono-Pen and pachymetry ($p = 0.022$). The thicker the cornea, the larger the difference between the Tono-Pen and Perkins.

A Williams-T-Test for comparing dependent correlations revealed that the correlation between pachymetry and the Tono-Pen was not significantly stronger than the one between pachymetry and iCare ($t(36) = -1.40$, $p = 0.170$), but it was significantly stronger than the correlation between pachymetry and Perkins ($t(36) = -2.30$, $p = 0.027$).

The Bland–Altmann test showed that the regression of the difference against the mean of the two methods had a significant slope, as can be seen in the comparison of iCare to Perkins (Figure 1a), the Tono-Pen to Perkins (Figure 1b), and iCare to the Tono-Pen (Figure 1c).

However, when excluding IOP values over 25 mmHg, the regression of the difference against the mean of the two methods did not show a significant slope (Figure 2a,b). This relationship is also illustrated by scatterplots showing the IOP readings from two devices for each study eye separately (Supplementary Figure S1a–c). Table 2 summarizes these findings.

Table 1. Demographic and clinical characteristics of the study population.

children (n)	19
female (n)	11
male (n)	8
age (years)	1.8 ± 2.08
eyes (n)	38
aphakia (n)	18
congenital cataract	10
congenital glaucoma	7
nystagmus and/or hyperopia	3
corneal diameter (mean ± SD; mm)	horizontal: 10.6 ± 1.4 vertical: 10.1 ± 1.5
corneal thickness (mean ± SD; μm)	all eyes: 645 ± 135 aphakic eyes: 733 ± 267 phakic eyes: 604 ± 351 eyes with glaucoma: 744 ± 224
IOP, all devices [mean ± SD, (range); mmHg]	14.1 ± 7.4 (5–43)
Perkins	11.1 ± 4.8 (5–34)
iCare	11.6 ± 4.4 (6.4–36.4)
Tono-Pen	15.2 ± 5.5 (7–37)

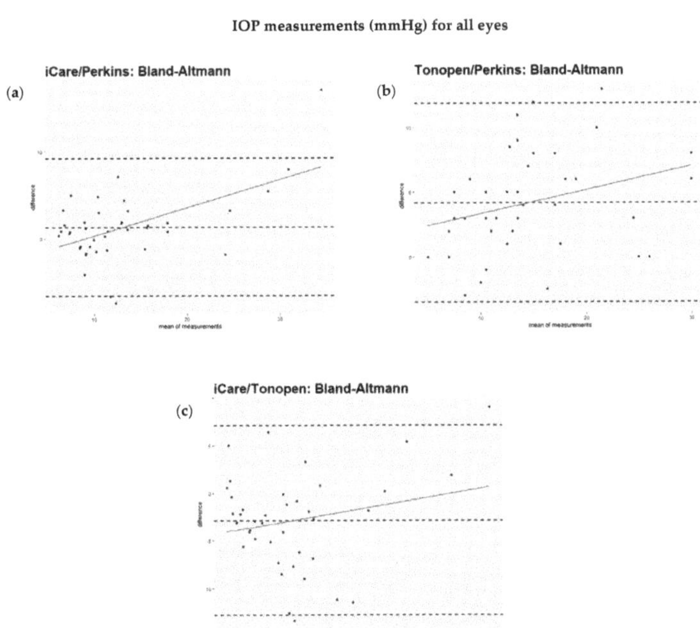

Figure 1. (**a–c**): Bland–Altmann analysis of intraocular pressure readings comparing different devices. All values are described in mmHg. (**a**): Bland–Altmann analysis comparing iCare and Perkins readings. The slope is positive (0.42). The result is highly significant ($p < 0.005$). (**b**): Analysis comparing Tono-Pen and Perkins readings. The slope is positive (0.2). The result is significant ($p = 0.04$). (**c**): Bland–Altmann analysis comparing iCare and Tono-Pen readings. The slope is positive (0.25). The p value is 0.02.

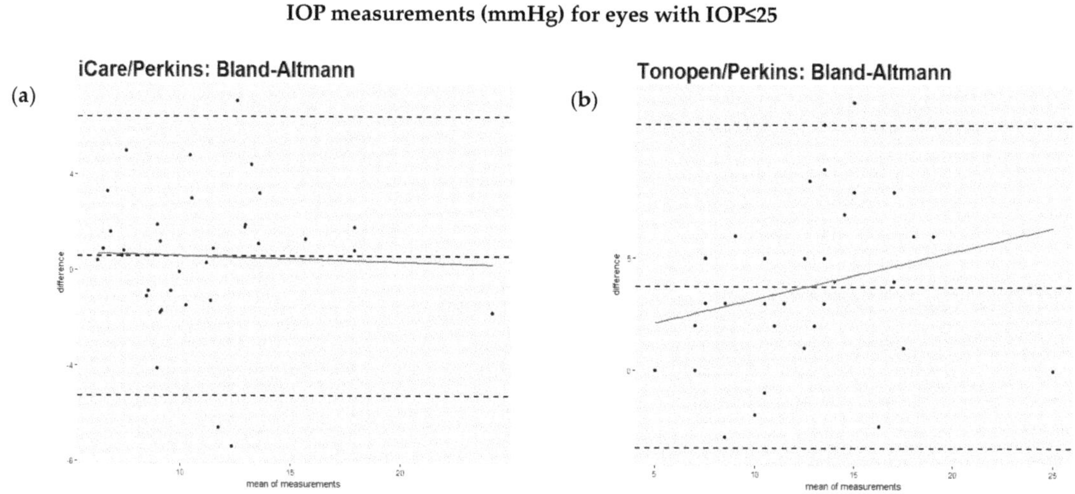

Figure 2. (**a**,**b**): Bland–Altmann analysis of intraocular pressure readings comparing different devices excluding measurements above 25 mmHg. All values are described in mmHg. (**a**): Bland–Altmann analysis comparing iCare and Perkins readings excluding measurements above 25 mmHg. When excluding readings above 25 mmHg, no significant difference between the two methods was found (regression slope = −0.12, p = 0.39). (**b**): Analysis comparing Tono-Pen and Perkins readings excluding measurements above 25 mmHg. When excluding readings above 25 mmHg, no significant difference was found between the two devices (regression slope = 0.2, p = 0.24).

Table 2. Bland–Altman regression analysis of the difference versus the mean for comparisons between Perkins, the Tono-Pen, and iCare. A significant positive slope indicates increasing disagreement with higher intraocular pressure (IOP). Results on the right show regressions after excluding IOP values >25 mmHg; none were statistically significant ($p > 0.05$).

Comparison Pair	Slope (All Values)	p-Value	Slope (IOP $\leq$ 25 mmHg)	p-Value
iCare vs. Perkins	0.42	<0.005	−0.12	0.39
Tono-Pen vs. Perkins	0.20	0.04	0.20	0.24
iCare vs. Tono-Pen	0.25	0.02	−0.30	0.15

4. Discussion

Measurement of the intraocular pressure with GAT is considered the gold standard. The iCare tonometer is based on the method of "rebound tonometry". The iCare tonometer enables non-invasive and well-tolerated IOP measurements in children without the need for topical anesthesia, making it particularly suitable for non-cooperative pediatric patients. Its implementation has substantially reduced the frequency of examinations under general anesthesia, especially for routine screening. These findings are in agreement with the study by Grigorian et al., which demonstrated a significant reduction in the number of examinations under anesthesia following the introduction of iCare [18].

The current study showed a good correlation between the rebound tonometer iCare and Perkins applanation handheld tonometer. This finding aligns with other studies reporting a good correlation between iCare and Perkins in children [21]. Borrego Sanz et al. reported a difference between these two tonometers in children with primary congenital glaucoma of 0.42 ± 3.69 mmHg, with higher iCare readings [22]. In another study of Martinez-de-la-Casa et al., the comparison between Perkins and iCare in congenital glaucoma also showed a good correlation with significantly higher readings in iCare (mean of 3.1 mmHg) [23].

In pediatric glaucoma with different corneal pathologies, Angmo et al. found a mean difference of 0.82 mmHg [24], and Umfress et al. found a mean difference of 1.2 mmHg [25]. Stoddard-Bennett et al. described in healthy children a mean difference of 0.72 mmHg with no influence of central corneal thickness [26].

Lambert et al. described in a review a good correlation between rebound tonometry and Goldman applanation tonometry with a higher reading in rebound tonometry of 2 to 3 mmHg higher in the 2 level II studies performed in a clinic setting and in 1 level III study performed on children under general anesthesia [21].

In our study, which included a variety of diagnoses and a higher number of aphakic eyes, no significant difference was observed between the iCare and the Perkins device (11.6 mmHg $\pm$ 4.4 vs. 11.1 $\pm$ 4.8 mmHg). This is noteworthy, as the mean corneal pachymetry in our cohort (mean 645.6 µm $\pm$ 135.4) was higher than in other studies, such as that by Martinez-de-la-Casa et al. (556.5 $\pm$ 56.1 µm) [23]. Higher IOP readings with iCare in thicker corneas have been documented in the literature [27], a finding confirmed in our study. Nevertheless, the difference between iCare and Perkins was small in this study. Esmael et al. reported a small but statistically significant difference of -0.59 ± 2.59 mmHg between rebound and applanation tonometry in children [28]. In our study, the mean difference was of similar magnitude (-0.5 mmHg), although it did not reach statistical significance. This may be attributed to the smaller sample size in our cohort. Moreover, while Esmael et al. observed declining agreement above 15 mmHg, our data indicate a more pronounced divergence above 25 mmHg, supporting the recommendation to confirm elevated IOP with Perkins applanation tonometry in clinical practice.

The thicker central corneal thickness in this study might be explained by the fact that a large number of patients with anterior segment abnormalities, notably aphakia, have been included. It has been shown that patients with aphakia and small cornea diameters have thicker corneas and therefore have a greater-than-normal measured IOP [29].

Consistent with the findings of Yulia et al. [30], our study confirms that rebound tonometry is a valuable tool for IOP screening in pediatric populations. Both studies reported an increasing discrepancy between rebound and applanation tonometry at higher IOP levels—above 25 mmHg in our cohort and above 19 mmHg in theirs. However, unlike Yulia et al. [30] who observed a tendency of rebound tonometry to overestimate IOP in children with congenital corneal opacities, we cannot evaluate this effect, as corneal opacity was an exclusion criterion in our study.

When we excluded IOP readings above 25 mmHg, the differences between the methods decreased. The slope of regression of the differences was no longer significant. The same applied to the regression of differences against pachymetry. A substantially higher deviation between devices in IOP readings above 22 mmHg has also been shown by others [31].

In this study, IOP readings were obtained under general anesthesia. It is known that anesthetic agents can alter IOP readings in a time-dependent manner [32,33]. However, this should not have a relevant influence on our results, primarily because the focus of this study focused on the difference between devices rather than absolute IO values, Moreover, all measurements were taken under the same conditions once sedation was effective within five minutes—an interval during which IOP is generally stable between minutes two and eight after anesthesia induction [33].

Study Limitations

Despite its strengths, this study has several limitations that should be considered. First, the relatively small sample size and the retrospective design may limit the generalizability of the findings. A larger cohort would increase statistical power and allow for more robust conclusions. Second, the inclusion of both eyes from individual patients may have introduced bias by duplicating anatomical or physiological characteristics that could influence IOP measurements in a similar way across both eyes. Third, the lack of randomization in both the order of eye measurements (always starting with the right eye) and the sequence of tonometer use may have introduced order-related bias. Fourth, as all measurements were performed by the same examiner, masking was not possible. These limitations should be taken into account when interpreting the results and underline the need for future prospective studies with randomized protocols and larger, controlled populations. Another limitation is the lack of blinding during the measurement process. In this study, the investigator had access to prior IOP readings from different devices, which could have introduced observer bias. Future studies should implement blinded measurement protocols, where examiners are unaware of previous results, to ensure greater objectivity and eliminate potential bias in data collection.

The diversity of diagnoses among the included patients also presents a challenge. While the variability of diagnosis reflects real-world clinical practice, it also complicates direct comparisons between different tonometry methods. Future research could benefit from more uniform patient selection criteria, focusing on specific subgroups to improve the accuracy of device comparisons.

Additionally, since all IOP measurements were conducted under general anesthesia, the potential effects of anesthetic agents on IOP values must be considered. Although the study standardized the timing of IOP measurements to minimize these effects, it remains possible that anesthesia altered the IOP readings to some extent. Nevertheless, further investigation is needed to assess the potential impact of different anesthetic agents on IOP readings obtained with various tonometry devices [34,35]. Another factor that may have influenced the findings is corneal thickness variability among the study participants. The mean corneal pachymetry in this study was higher than in previous research, and it has been established in the literature that iCare tonometry tends to overestimate IOP in thicker corneas [36]. Since this study included patients with a higher-than-average corneal thickness, the degree of overestimation by iCare could have been more pronounced compared to other studies with thinner corneas. This should be taken into account when interpreting the results and when selecting a tonometer for pediatric patients with variable corneal properties.

Given these limitations, future research should focus on larger, prospective, multicenter studies including matched controls to improve statistical reliability and ensure a more diverse and representative patient population. Implementing blinded measurement protocols and ensuring a more homogeneous study cohort would further enhance the accuracy of findings. By addressing these limitations, future studies can provide a clearer and more definitive understanding of the performance of different tonometers in pediatric patients under general anesthesia.

5. Conclusions

This study aimed to compare Goldmann applanation tonometry (Perkins), iCare rebound tonometry, and the Tono-Pen in young children undergoing examination under general anesthesia. All patients were suspected of elevated IOP, making this a rare and clinically important study population.

Our findings suggest that the Perkins tonometer remains the preferred device in young patients under general anesthesia, particularly when IOP exceeds 25 mmHg or corneal thickness is abnormally high. For children with normal corneal thickness and IOP values equal or below 25 mmHg, the iCare tonometer proved to be a reliable alternative, offering ease of use and less operator dependency.

The Tono-Pen exhibited significant deviations, consistently overestimating IOP compared to Perkins, thus limiting its reliability in pediatric glaucoma evaluation under general anesthesia.

Overall, this study highlights the importance of selecting the most appropriate tonometry device for pediatric patients, particularly those requiring examination under anesthesia. Future research should aim to validate these findings in larger, multicenter trials, ensuring greater statistical power and improved generalizability.

Supplementary Materials: The following supporting information can be downloaded at https://www.mdpi.com/article/10.3390/jcm14103338/s1. Figure S1. Scatterplots showing intraocular pressure (IOP) measurements of two tonometry devices for each study eye. Each point pair on the x-axis represents one study eye, with corresponding IOP values from the two compared devices plotted on the y-axis. As demonstrated by Bland-Altman analysis (Figures 1 and 2), best agreement is observed between iCare and Perkins after excluding IOP values above 25 mmHg.

Author Contributions: Conceptualization, B.E.F. and S.A.F.; Methodology, M.I., B.E.F. and S.A.F.; Validation, C.T.; Formal analysis, M.K.S. and S.A.F.; Investigation, M.K.S.; Writing—original draft, M.K.S.; Writing—review & editing, M.I., C.T., B.E.F. and S.A.F. All authors have read and agreed to the published version of the manuscript.

Funding: This research received no external funding.

Institutional Review Board Statement: The study was approved by the Swissethics, Kantonale Ethikkommission Bern, code, BASEC-Nr: 2020-00635; approved date 29 January 2023.

Informed Consent Statement: Informed consent was obtained from all subjects involved in the study.

Data Availability Statement: The raw data supporting the conclusions of this article will be made available by the authors on request.

Conflicts of Interest: The authors declare no conflicts of interest.

References

1. Kass, M.A.; Heuer, D.K.; Higginbotham, E.J.; Johnson, C.A.; Keltner, J.L.; Miller, J.P.; Parrish, R.K., 2nd; Wilson, M.R.; Gordon, M.O. The Ocular Hypertension Treatment Study: A randomized trial determines that topical ocular hypotensive medication delays or prevents the onset of primary open-angle glaucoma. *Arch. Ophthalmol.* **2002**, *120*, 701–713. [CrossRef] [PubMed]
2. Leske, M.C.; Heijl, A.; Hyman, L.; Bengtsson, B. Early Manifest Glaucoma Trial: Design and baseline data. *Ophthalmology* **1999**, *106*, 2144–2153. [CrossRef] [PubMed]
3. Chagny, M.; Stolowy, N.; Denis, D.; Sauvan, L. Comparison of the iCare rebound tonometer and the Perkins applanation tonometer in children under general anesthesia. *J. Français D'ophtalmologie* **2023**, *46*, 1005–1012. [CrossRef]
4. Ko, F.; Papadopoulos, M.; Khaw, P.T. Primary congenital glaucoma. *Prog. Brain Res.* **2015**, *221*, 177–189. [CrossRef] [PubMed]
5. Yassin, S.A. Long-Term Visual Outcomes in Children with Primary Congenital Glaucoma. *Eur. J. Ophthalmol.* **2017**, *27*, 705–710. [CrossRef]
6. Strzalkowska, A.; Pirlich, N.; Stingl, J.V.; Schuster, A.K.; Rezapour, J.; Wagner, F.M.; Buse, J.; Hoffmann, E.M. Intraocular Pressure Measurement in Childhood Glaucoma under Standardized General Anaesthesia: The Prospective EyeBIS Study. *J. Clin. Med.* **2022**, *11*, 2846. [CrossRef]
7. Feng, C.S.; Jin, K.W.; Yi, K.; Choi, D.G. Comparison of Intraocular Pressure Measurements Obtained by Rebound, Noncontact, and Goldmann Applanation Tonometry in Children. *Am. J. Ophthalmol.* **2015**, *160*, 937–943 e931. [CrossRef]
8. Krieglstein, G.K.; Waller, W.K. Goldmann applanation versus hand-applanation and .schiotz indentation tonometry. *Albrecht Graefes Arch. Klin. Exp. Ophthalmol.* **1975**, *194*, 11–16. [CrossRef]

9. Browning, A.C.; Bhan, A.; Rotchford, A.P.; Shah, S.; Dua, H.S. The effect of corneal thickness on intraocular pressure measurement in patients with corneal pathology. *Br. J. Ophthalmol.* **2004**, *88*, 1395–1399. [CrossRef]
10. McKee, E.C.; Ely, A.L.; Duncan, J.E.; Dosunmu, E.O.; Freedman, S.F. A comparison of Icare PRO and Tono-Pen XL tonometers in anesthetized children. *J. Am. Assoc. Pediatr. Ophthalmol. Strabismus* **2015**, *19*, 332–337. [CrossRef]
11. Hsiao, Y.C.; Dzau, J.R.; Flemmons, M.S.; Asrani, S.; Jones, S.; Freedman, S.F. Home assessment of diurnal intraocular pressure in healthy children using the Icare rebound tonometer. *J. Am. Assoc. Pediatr. Ophthalmol. Strabismus* **2012**, *16*, 58–60. [CrossRef] [PubMed]
12. Boothe, W.A.; Lee, D.A.; Panek, W.C.; Pettit, T.H. The Tono-Pen. A manometric and clinical study. *Arch. Ophthalmol.* **1988**, *106*, 1214–1217. [CrossRef]
13. Yildiz, M.B.; Kose, A.O.; Celik, G.; Kizilay, O.; Imamoglu, S.; Yildiz, E. Agreement among Goldmann Applanation Tonometer, Easyton Transpalpebral Tonometer, Tonopen, and Icare in Patients with Keratoconus. *Beyoglu Eye J.* **2023**, *8*, 170–176. [CrossRef] [PubMed]
14. Tayar, A.; Grossjohann, R.; Stahl, A.; Tost, F. Comparing Different Self-Tonometry Devices against Goldmann Applanation Tonometry—Special Focus on Biomechanical Properties of the Cornea. *Klin. Monbl. Augenheilkd* **2025**, *242*, 137–145. [CrossRef]
15. Kontiola, A.; Puska, P. Measuring intraocular pressure with the Pulsair 3000 and Rebound tonometers in elderly patients without an anesthetic. *Graefes Arch. Clin. Exp. Ophthalmol.* **2004**, *242*, 3–7. [CrossRef] [PubMed]
16. Mendez-Hernandez, C.; Arribas-Pardo, P.; Sanchez Jean, R.; Garcia-Feljoo, J. Influence of Axial Length on Intraocular Pressure Measurement With Three Tonometers in Childhood Glaucoma. *J. Pediatr. Ophthalmol. Strabismus* **2020**, *57*, 27–32. [CrossRef]
17. Karhanova, M.; Kalitova, J.; Maluskova, M.; Schovanek, J.; Zapletalova, J.; Mlcak, P.; Maresova, K. Comparison of Three Methods of Tonometry in Patients with Inactive Thyroid-Associated Orbitopathy. *Cesk Slov. Oftalmol.* **2023**, *79*, 318–323. [CrossRef]
18. Grigorian, F.; Grigorian, A.P.; Olitsky, S. The Effect of Introduction of iCare Tonometer in the Pediatric Ophthalmology Clinic on Number of Examinations Under Anesthesia. *Investig. Ophthalmol. Vis. Sci.* **2011**, *52*, 679.
19. Duran, M. Comparison of intraocular pressure measurements obtained by icare pro tonometer, non-contact tonometer and Goldmann applanation tonometer in healthy individuals. *J. Français D'ophtalmologie* **2023**, *46*, 1195–1203. [CrossRef]
20. Liu, J.; Roberts, C.J. Influence of corneal biomechanical properties on intraocular pressure measurement: Quantitative analysis. *J. Cataract. Refract. Surg.* **2005**, *31*, 146–155. [CrossRef]
21. Lambert, S.R.; Melia, M.; Buffenn, A.N.; Chiang, M.F.; Simpson, J.L.; Yang, M.B. Rebound tonometry in children: A report by the American Academy of Ophthalmology. *Ophthalmology* **2013**, *120*, e21–e27. [CrossRef]
22. Borrego Sanz, L.; Morales-Fernandez, L.; Martinez de-la-Casa, J.M.; Saenz-Frances, F.; Fuentes, M.; Garcia-Feijoo, J. The Icare-Pro Rebound Tonometer Versus the Hand-held Applanation Tonometer in Congenital Glaucoma. *J. Glaucoma* **2016**, *25*, 149–154. [CrossRef] [PubMed]
23. Martinez-de-la-Casa, J.M.; Garcia-Feijoo, J.; Saenz-Frances, F.; Vizzeri, G.; Fernandez-Vidal, A.; Mendez-Hernandez, C.; Garcia-Sanchez, J. Comparison of rebound tonometer and Goldmann handheld applanation tonometer in congenital glaucoma. *J. Glaucoma* **2009**, *18*, 49–52. [CrossRef]
24. Angmo, D.; Ramesh, P.; Mahalingam, K.; Azmira, K.; Pandey, S.; Gupta, V.; Sihota, R.; Dada, T. Comparative Evaluation of Rebound and Perkins Tonometers in Pediatric Glaucoma With Varied Corneal Characteristics. *J. Glaucoma* **2021**, *30*, 312–316. [CrossRef]
25. Umfress, A.C.; Glaser, T.S.; Ploysangam, P.; Freedman, S.F. Rebound tonometry by iCare 200 (IC200): Comparison with Tono-Pen in the operating room and Goldmann applanation in the clinic. *J. Am. Assoc. Pediatr. Ophthalmol. Strabismus* **2021**, *25*, 329 e321–329 e326. [CrossRef] [PubMed]
26. Stoddard-Bennett, T.; Jackson, N.J.; Robbins, L.; Villanueva, P.; Suh, S.Y.; Demer, J.L.; Pineles, S.L.; Fung, S.S.M. Agreement of iCare IC200 tonometry with Perkins applanation tonometry in healthy children. *J. Am. Assoc. Pediatr. Ophthalmol. Strabismus* **2022**, *26*, 235 e231–235 e235. [CrossRef] [PubMed]
27. Poostchi, A.; Mitchell, R.; Nicholas, S.; Purdie, G.; Wells, A. The iCare rebound tonometer: Comparisons with Goldmann tonometry, and influence of central corneal thickness. *Clin. Exp. Ophthalmol.* **2009**, *37*, 687–691. [CrossRef]
28. Esmael, A.; Ismail, Y.M.; Elhusseiny, A.M.; Fayed, A.E.; Elhilali, H.M. Agreement profiles for rebound and applanation tonometry in normal and glaucomatous children. *Eur. J. Ophthalmol.* **2019**, *29*, 379–385. [CrossRef]
29. Bayoumi, N.H.; El Shakankiri, N.M. Central Corneal Thickness in Aphakic Children With Microcornea-Microphthalmia. *J. Glaucoma* **2016**, *25*, 497–500. [CrossRef]
30. Yulia, D.E.; Tan, S. Intraocular pressure measurements in paediatric glaucoma: A narrative review on accuracy, tolerability, and ease of use. *Med. J. Malays.* **2024**, *79*, 206–211.

31. Munkwitz, S.; Elkarmouty, A.; Hoffmann, E.M.; Pfeiffer, N.; Thieme, H. Comparison of the iCare rebound tonometer and the Goldmann applanation tonometer over a wide IOP range. *Graefes Arch. Clin. Exp. Ophthalmol.* **2008**, *246*, 875–879. [CrossRef] [PubMed]
32. Jones, L.; Sung, V.; Lascaratos, G.; Nagi, H.; Holder, R. Intraocular pressures after ketamine and sevoflurane in children with glaucoma undergoing examination under anaesthesia. *Br. J. Ophthalmol.* **2010**, *94*, 33–35. [CrossRef] [PubMed]
33. Blumberg, D.; Congdon, N.; Jampel, H.; Gilbert, D.; Elliott, R.; Rivers, R.; Munoz, B.; Quigley, H. The effects of sevoflurane and ketamine on intraocular pressure in children during examination under anesthesia. *Am. J. Ophthalmol.* **2007**, *143*, 494–499. [CrossRef]
34. Oatts, J.T.; Shen, S.; Zhu, H.; Gong, Q.; Yu, Y.; Ying, G.S.; Han, Y.; Liu, H. A Prospective Study of the Effects of General Anesthesia on Intraocular Pressure in Healthy Children. *Ophthalmol. Sci.* **2024**, *4*, 100455. [CrossRef] [PubMed]
35. Senthil, S.; Nakka, M.; Rout, U.; Ali, H.; Choudhari, N.; Badakere, S.; Garudadri, C. Changes in intraocular pressures associated with inhalational and mixed anesthetic agents currently used in ophthalmic surgery. *Indian J. Ophthalmol.* **2021**, *69*, 1808–1814. [CrossRef]
36. Rao, A.; Kumar, M.; Prakash, B.; Varshney, G. Relationship of central corneal thickness and intraocular pressure by iCare rebound tonometer. *J. Glaucoma* **2014**, *23*, 380–384. [CrossRef]

Journal of
Clinical Medicine

MDPI

Article

Affordable Sinskey Hook Goniotomy and Cataract Surgery in Black and Afro-Latino Patients Diagnosed with Glaucoma: Retrospective Real-World One-Year Results

Idaima Calderon [1] and Daniel Laroche [1,2,*]

[1] Advanced Eyecare of New York, New York, NY 10027, USA; idaima.calderon@gmail.com
[2] New York Eye and Ear of Mount Sinai, New York, NY 10027, USA
* Correspondence: dlarochemd@aol.com; Tel.: +1-212-663-0473

Abstract: Background/Objectives: This study aimed to evaluate the effectiveness of early phacoemulsification cataract surgery combined with goniotomy using a Sinskey hook in patients with glaucoma. **Methods**: This was a retrospective study conducted at Advanced Eye Care of New York; a private practice located in New York City. Most patients carried diagnoses of mild to moderate glaucoma and were mainly Black and Afro-Latino in origin. The patients included in this study were those who underwent early phacoemulsification cataract surgery combined with goniotomy performed with a reusable Sinskey hook (Ambler 200 µm tip) between January 2022 and August 2023 and completed 1 year of follow-up. The primary outcome measures were intraocular pressure, number of medications used, visual acuity, visual field indices, pre-/post-operative spherical refractive error, and adverse events. **Results**: A total of 121 eyes were identified with a 1-year follow-up that underwent this combined surgery. The mean age was 65. The mean medically treated pre-operative intraocular pressure $\pm$ standard deviation (SD) was lowered from 16.40 $\pm$ 4.5 mmHg at baseline to 14.66 $\pm$ 3.1 mmHg at 1 year, a statistically significant reduction of 10.6%. There was an 82% reduction in the mean $\pm$ SD number of intraocular pressure-lowering medications used, from 1.67 $\pm$ 1.2 at baseline to 0.30 $\pm$ 0.8 at 1 year. Out of the 121 eyes, 83% (103 eyes) remained medication-free at 1-year post-operation. Post-operatively, there were five IOP spikes (IOP $\geq$ 30 mmHg) and eight hyphemas that were noted, addressed, and resolved. **Conclusions**: Early cataract surgery combined with Sinskey hook goniotomy microinvasive surgery effectively reduced intraocular pressure and medication burden in this cohort of predominantly Black and Afro-Latino patients diagnosed with glaucoma with 1-year follow-up.

Keywords: Sinskey hook; goniotomy; MIGS; glaucoma

1. Introduction

Glaucoma is the leading cause of preventable blindness globally and disproportionally affects Black and Afro-Latino populations [1]. A 2024 meta-analysis estimates that glaucoma affects over 4 million people in the US and is 2–3 times more prevalent in Black adults than their White counterparts [1]. Other studies approximate the rate is closer to 3–4 times greater [2]. Increased intraocular pressure (IOP) is the primary risk factor for glaucoma and the main target in treatment [3]. Though the mean IOP in the general population is estimated to be approximately 15 mm Hg, prior studies have found mean pressures in untreated glaucomatous eyes often range from 18 mm Hg to mid-low 20 s [2,3]. The current therapeutic options to reduce IOP include medications, laser surgery, and incisional procedures. Though eye pressure-lowering medications are an effective way to reduce eye pressure and slow the progression of the disease, they can be limited in their ability to completely halt progression [4,5]. Factors such as suboptimal medication adherence (missed doses) and diminished persistence (continued use of medication over time) are associated with worsening visual field (VF) progression and are problems that disproportionately affect high-risk sociodemographic groups [4–6]. Health disparities like these are more likely to affect Black and Afro-Latino communities, as these populations often face greater barriers and inequities related to socioeconomic status, education, language fluency, health literacy, insurance coverage, and access to care, and are a byproduct of a greater historical context and systemic issues [6–11].

Early cataract surgery combined with trabecular bypass surgery represents a viable alternative intervention that effectively lowers intraocular pressure (IOP) and reduces reliance on medications. This approach merits consideration as a first-line strategy for patients aged 50 and above diagnosed with glaucoma- and age-related lens enlargement, particularly when performed by skilled surgeons [9]. Cataract and age-related increases in lens size and thickness can play a major role in glaucoma through mechanisms such as pupillary block and by contributing to pigment liberation through iridolenticular contact and the obstruction of the trabecular meshwork [9]. Cataract surgery has been proven to safely and effectively lower IOP by 13–71% in patients with comorbid open- or closed-angle glaucoma [9,12–15]. The EAGLE study [14] found early lens extraction to be more effective than laser iridotomy in treating angle closure glaucoma and recommended it as a first-line treatment. Early cataract surgery and goniotomy have also been shown to be efficacious in patients with open-angle glaucoma [16–19]. As glaucoma within the Black population has been shown to present at earlier ages and with more advanced disease and complications [7,8,18], early surgical intervention could help prevent vision loss and circumvent challenges related to medication adherence.

In recent years, minimally invasive glaucoma surgery (MIGS) has emerged as a widely adopted alternative for treating mild to moderate glaucoma, though the high cost of these devices remains a challenge. However, the high cost associated with using these devices [19,20] can limit their access and use in lower resource areas around the world. Several studies have attempted to shed light on more affordable MIGS options: one reported the Kahook Dual Blade as the most cost-effective device [20] and other studies have reported on more affordable surgical alternatives that use comparable techniques, such as goniotomy with a Tanito hook [19–21].

Previously, we reported our preliminary data using another inexpensive device to perform MIGS in conjunction with cataract surgery, the Sinskey hook [19]. We commented on the advantage of the Sinskey hook's 200-μm tip size and smoothness, which corresponded well with the size of the trabecular meshwork and reduced the potential of bleeding from injury to the ciliary body or the back wall of Schlemm's canal. Our preliminary findings suggested that cataract extraction paired with goniotomy using the Sinskey hook was an affordable and effective method to lower IOP and medication burden in Black and Afro-Latino patients diagnosed with glaucoma. This report aims to provide one-year surgical outcomes of patients who underwent cataract surgery with goniotomy using the Sinskey hook.

2. Materials and Methods

This retrospective single-center analysis examines surgical outcomes in a predominantly Black and Afro-Latino (self-identified) patient population with glaucoma who received combined phacoemulsification cataract surgery and goniotomy utilizing a 200 μm tip Sinskey hook (Ambler Surgical, Exton, PA, USA). Patients of all races who carried a diagnosis of mild to moderate open-angle or narrow-angle glaucoma and who underwent this procedure between January 2022 and August 2023 and had completed 1-year follow-up were included in this study. Patients with severe glaucoma and/or synechial angle closure were not offered this procedure and were, thus, excluded. Retrospective patient data were collected from a private practice located in Harlem, New York City, USA, and Queens Village, NY, USA. Glaucoma subtypes were noted.

Informed consent was waived due to the retrospective nature of the study, as approved by the Icahn School of Medicine of Mount Sinai Institutional Review Board (IRB). The study was conducted in accordance with the Declaration of Helsinki.

Data were obtained throughout the clinical course of each patient, at their pre-operative visit and their post-operative visits at one day, one month, six months, and one year following surgery. The goal was to significantly reduce intraocular pressure and the amount of medication needed in all the included patients, as compared to baseline. However, the medical needs, target intraocular pressure, and baseline pressure measurements were varied and specific to each individual patient. As such, the decision to restart or eliminate medication was assessed during patient follow-up visits and then performed as clinically indicated.

A reusable, straight Sinskey hook, an instrument commonly used in cataract surgery, was utilized to open the trabecular meshwork and the inner wall of Schlemm's canal. This ophthalmic tool leaves a 200 μm wide opening and reduces bleeding risk, due to the blunt tip and smooth back end of the device. The device was reused several times without any noted difference in efficacy. If the device were to become damaged during sterilization or other handling, then a new one would be used. A total of four devices were used between four operating rooms, with one replaced due to damage to the tip during sterilization.

The study's primary outcome measures included intraocular pressure, amount of medication used, best corrected visual acuity (BCVA) pre-/post-operatively, visual field, pre-/post-operative spherical refractive error, and adverse events. Humphrey Visual Field Analyzer (Zeiss Humphrey Systems, San Leandro, CA, USA) 24-2 results were reviewed before the surgery and at 1 year post-operation. Target post-operative refraction was between 0 to −0.5 diopters by ocular biometry.

Procedure

The patients were administered a pre-operative regimen of prednisolone acetate 1% (Allergan, Dublin, Ireland) four times daily (QID), ofloxacin (Rising, Saddle Brook, NJ, USA) QID, and Ketorolac 0.4% (Allergan, Dublin, Ireland) three times daily (TID), starting 3 days prior to surgery. Preparations for the eye on the day of surgery included betadine and draping, and the application of topical anesthesia. Phacoemulsification cataract surgery was performed through a clear cornea, and an intraocular lens was implanted. To deepen the angle, EndoCoat (Abbott, Chicago, IL, USA) was injected into the anterior chamber and on the cornea. To optimize visualization, adjustments were then made to tilt the patient's head to approximately 45° away from the surgeon, while the microscope was tilted toward the surgeon at the same angle. Structures in the nasal angle were visualized after focusing the microscope through a direct gonio lens (Katena, Troy Hills, NJ, USA) that was positioned on top of the eye. A Microvitreoretinal (MVR) blade was then utilized to penetrate the trabecular meshwork and create an opening in Schlemm's canal. Following this, a Sinskey hook was introduced into Schlemm's canal and passed approximately 2–3 clock hours to the left and then to the right to unroof the canal (Figure 1). After completing this step, the

Sinskey hook was withdrawn and balanced salt solution was injected via paracentesis, and the wound was hydrated and closed pressurizing the eye to about 20 mmHG. At the conclusion of the procedure, an intracameral injection of diluted Vigamox (Alcon, Geneva, Switzerland) mixed in a 50/50 ratio with a balanced saline solution was administered via paracentesis. It was observed that in all the patients, the nasal angle remained open following cataract surgery. The corneal incisions were hydrated and sealed effectively to ensure no leakage. Post-operatively, the patients were immediately placed in a seated position to keep their heads elevated above waist level to reduce episcleral venous pressure.

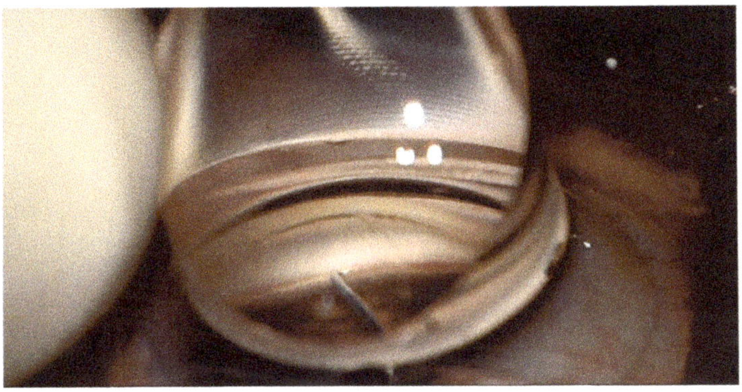

Figure 1. Goniotomy using a Sinskey hook.

The patients received instructions to sleep in an elevated position for four nights post-operatively to facilitate the settling and clearing of any potential heme reflux that could cause visual obstruction. They were advised to continue using ofloxacin QID for seven days. Prednisolone acetate 1% was tapered over four weeks (QID to TID to BID to daily—each dose taken for seven days) before discontinuation. Ketorolac 0.4% was continued TID for four weeks before being discontinued. The patients were also instructed to discontinue all glaucoma medications in the operated eye immediately after surgery. This comprehensive protocol ensured proper healing while optimizing surgical outcomes and maintaining intraocular pressure control.

3. Results

Of the participants who underwent phacoemulsification cataract extraction combined with a Sinskey hook goniotomy procedure and completed a 1-year follow-up, there were 121 eyes identified and enrolled in the study. The mean age of the participants was 65 ± 10 years, and 70% were female and 30% were male (Table 1). The self-described race and ethnicity demographics of our study population were 87% Black or Latino, 4% Non-Hispanic White, and 9% Asian (Table 2). Fifty (41%) participants were diagnosed with primary open-angle glaucoma, twenty-eight (23%) with ocular hypertension, twenty-four (20%) with angle-closure glaucoma, nine (7%) were glaucoma suspects, seven (6%) had narrow angles, and three (2%) had pigmentary glaucoma. All the baseline characteristics and calculations were collected on medically treated eyes, and included IOP, number of ocular hypertensive medications used, BCVA, and visual field index (VFI) and mean deviation (MD) on visual field test (VFT) (Table 1).

A statistically significant decrease in mean IOP for all the eyes was achieved following the phacoemulsification cataract surgery with Sinskey hook goniotomy at one-year follow-up (Table 3). The baseline mean pre-operative IOP and standard deviation for all the eyes was 16.40 ± 4.5 mmHg. As our study did not conduct a pre-operative washout of medications, our population started at a relatively lower baseline IOP. Nevertheless, on post-operative day 1, the mean IOP and standard deviation for all eyes were significantly lowered to 14.31 ± 6.2. This statistically significant reduction in IOP remained at one year, with the mean IOP and standard deviation for all the eyes at 14.66 ± 3.1 mmHg. This is a 10.6% reduction from baseline.

Table 1. Baseline characteristics of participants.

Variable	Category	Statistics, n Total = 121
Age (years)	Mean ± SD	65 ± 10.4
Gender, n (%)	Female	85 (71%)
	Male	36 (30%)
Eye, n (%)	Right	66 (55%)
	Left	55 (45%)
Baseline IOP (mmHg)	Mean ± SD	16.40 ± 4.5
Ocular hypertensive medications	Mean ± SD	1.67 ± 1.2
Number of ocular hypertensive medications used, (%)	0	17 (14%)
	1	57 (47%)
	2	8 (7%)
	3	27 (22%)
	≥4	12 (10%)
Visual acuity (logMar)	Mean ± SD	0.37 ± 0.3
MD on VFT	Mean ± SD	−6.63 ± 7.0
VFI on VFT	Mean ± SD	86.2% ± 20.2

Table 2. Race and ethnic origin of participants.

	N Total = 121
Black, n (%)	103 (85%)
White, n (%)	7 (6%)
Asian, n (%)	11 (9%)
Hispanic, total, n (%)	15 (12%)
Hispanic, Black, n (%)	13 (11%)
Hispanic, White, n (%)	2 (2%)
Non-Hispanic, White only, n (%)	5 (4%)

Table 3. Post-operative data for all patients who underwent phacoemulsification cataract surgery with Sinskey hook goniotomy.

Timepoint	Intraocular Pressure (IOP) mmHG, Mean ± SD	Ocular Hypertensive Medications, Mean ± SD	BCVA logMAR, Mean ± SD	Visual Field Test, Mean Deviation ± SD
Baseline	16.40 ± 4.5	1.67 ± 1.2	0.37 ± 0.3	−6.63 ± 7.0
Post-operative day 1	14.31 * ± 6.2	0 *	-	
1 month	15.96 ± 4.8	0.18 * ± 0.7	0.13 ± 0.3	
3 months	13.87 * ± 4.4	0.27 * ± 0.8	0.11 ± 0.2	
6 months	14.27 * ± 3.2	0.30 * ± 0.8	0.11 ± 0.3	
1 year	14.66 * ± 3.1	0.30 * ± 0.8	0.12 ± 0.3	−5.48 ± 6.1

* Statistically significant reduction from baseline.

At baseline, 86% (104 out of 121 eyes) were taking intraocular pressure-lowering medications. The mean ± standard deviation number of pressure-lowering medications used for all the eyes at baseline was 1.67 ± 1.2. At 1-year, we observed a statistically significant decrease to 0.30 ± 0.8, an 82% reduction. Out of the 121 eyes, 83% (103 eyes) remained medication-free at 1 year post-operation.

There was an improvement in the visual acuity and visual field measurements in mean totals from the baseline to the one-year follow-up. The mean BCVA (logMAR) and standard deviation in all the eyes improved from 0.37 ± 0.3 at baseline to 0.12 ± 0.3 at one year post-operation. There was a slight decrease in the mean spherical equivalent in all the eyes (Table 4) due to several outliers in the baseline data, which is reflected in the wider standard deviation. The mean pre-operative VFI% and MD in all the eyes were 86.2% and −6.63, respectively. The mean post-operative VFI% and MD in all the eyes were 89.0% and −5.48, respectively. Post-operatively, there were five IOP spikes (IOP ≥ 30 mmHg) that were treated and eight hyphemas that were noted, addressed, and resolved. All the complications were treated in the usual manner and resolved within a few days to two weeks.

Table 4. Mean spherical equivalents (SEs) for all eyes included.

	Mean Spherical Equivalent ± SD
Pre-operative SE for all eyes	−0.19 ± 3.51
Post-operative SE for all eyes	−0.53 ± 0.90

4. Discussion

This study shows that our surgical approach of early cataract surgery combined with Sinskey hook goniotomy was effective in improving visual acuity, reducing intraocular pressure, and decreasing medication burden one year following surgery. We found that our technique demonstrated a relatively favorable safety profile, with only a few minor adverse effects, all of which resolved without sequelae.

Cataract surgery paired with goniotomy should be considered at earlier stages of mild-to-moderate glaucoma and as an initial intervention for patients aged 50+ with glaucoma related to lens enlargement. Though IOP-lowering drops are effective in slowing disease progression, their effects are limited by the patient's ability to adhere to the medication regimen consistently over time. With studies estimating that at least 50% of the patients in the US are missing doses [4], it is important to explore alternative treatment options that can provide stable IOP reduction without facing the same vulnerabilities to external variables (such as medication costs, side effects, and confusion about regimen). The recent focus on MIGS provides a path for just that, with many studies demonstrating these new approaches and devices to be effective in the reduction in IOP and in the management of glaucoma, especially when paired with cataract surgery [13,22–24].

Consistent with this growing body of literature, our surgical approach was able to achieve and sustain similar levels of IOP control as other MIGS devices. One recent systematic review analyzed the clinical outcomes of MIGS devices with and without cataract surgery in 74 studies and reported that mean IOP at 12 months ranged between 11.4 and 18.1 mmHg [24], which is aligned with our result of 14.7 mmHg. Our results are also consistent with several studies that reported the 12-month outcomes of the Kahook Dual Blade with cataract surgery and showed mean IOPs ranging between 12.4 and 15.4 mmHg [25–27]. Although the 10.6% IOP reduction in our study is modest, this statistically significant reduction also holds clinical significance in that the lower IOP and decreased diurnal fluctuation reduce the risk of glaucoma progression in this population. Additionally, recent clinical trials have demonstrated that these reductions in IOP with MIGS can be sustainable in even longer terms. The largest prospective randomized clinical trial in MIGS, the HORIZON trial, has published the results for the Hydrus Microstent showing that IOP reduction was improved with combined surgery and maintained over 5 years, with many not requiring additional pharmacological therapy [22].

Similarly, the outcomes of our study demonstrated that combined cataract surgery with Sinskey hook goniotomy reduced medication burden by 82%, with 83% of the patients remaining medication free at one year. Glaucoma medication adherence and persistence rates in the US are suboptimal and can be influenced by factors such as medication costs, side effects, limited health literacy, access to care, and interference with quality of life, among many others [4,5,28]. Since lower adherence rates are associated with increased visual field progression [4,5], offering an early surgical treatment alternative in populations that are disproportionately affected by these challenges could help address some of these disparities, reduce disease burden, and help preserve vision. Our findings reinforce this argument and align with the other MIGS literature [24], in that we observed no deterioration in the post-operative visual field of our patients, suggesting a reduction in visual field progression.

One of the frequently reported advantages of MIGS devices is that they generally have better safety profiles than trabeculectomy and require less invasive surgery [13,22–24]. The added benefit of performing a goniotomy with the Sinskey hook is that it does not carry the same potential risk of complications that can occur with permanently implanted MIGS devices, such as malposition, migration, and obstruction [29]. Furthermore, the smooth tip of the Sinskey hook protects the back wall of Schlemm's canal and the 200 μm width fits nicely within the canal, allowing one to open it bluntly and in a circumferential manner. Only four clock hours are needed to open the canal to obtain efficacy and reduce complications of bleeding that can occur from sharper devices, such as a bent cystotome or needle goniotomy.

Further distinguishing the Sinskey hook is that it is a more affordable option that offers results comparable to other excisional goniotomy devices and MIGS. In a study conducted by Sood and Chen [20], a cost analysis was performed comparing the affordability of different MIGS in relation to their efficacy in reducing IOP (cost per mmHg of intraocular pressure reduction). The devices all performed similarly in efficacy; however, they found that cost-effectiveness was best in the Kahook Dual Blade, followed by the Hydrus Microstent, Trabectome, and then iStent Inject [20]. The Sinskey hook has shown similar results in regard to efficacy, but is even less expensive than the Kahook Dual Blade and Tanito hook. Since the direct costs of glaucoma care correlate strongly with disease severity, the Sinskey hook provides a cost-effective treatment option [30].

As an affordable alternative to other microinvasive surgical techniques, this approach carries important implications for patients in resource-poor areas in that it reduces barriers to care and increases accessibility to glaucoma surgical treatment. Low-resource regions of the world with a significant glaucoma burden, such as sub-Saharan Africa, Southeast Asia, and the Caribbean, often face increased rates of blindness from glaucoma [31,32]. This can be due to factors such as lack of access to care, challenges with medication adherence, and costs of treatment [31,32]. A recent cross-sectional study collected data from 10 sub-Saharan African countries and found that the most common reasons for patients to decline surgical intervention were fear and the cost of treatment [32]. The Sinskey hook is easily accessible, often coming in cataract surgical sets, and its reusability also makes it an ideal surgical alternative that could lower financial barriers to treatment for these patients. With its enhanced safety profile, this procedure provides hesitant patients an alternative means to avoid more invasive interventions, such as trabeculectomy.

Comparable outcomes may be observed with earlier manual small-incision cataract surgery (MSICS), where lens removal is performed in glaucoma patients. A study conducted in the Congo reported a 37.39% reduction in intraocular pressure (IOP) following MSICS in glaucomatous patients, with pre-operative IOP decreasing from 23.16 ± 5.68 mmHg to 14.5 ± 2.7 mmHg post-operatively. Further research should assess whether early MSICS alone or combined with Sinskey hook goniotomy offers greater efficacy for mild to moderate glaucoma cases [33]. Offering earlier, safer, more affordable surgery that reduces the need for long-term topical treatment would help address many of the barriers mentioned in this article and decrease the risk of disease progression. This should be performed by experienced surgeons. According to the 2023 data from the Association of American Medical Colleges (AAMC), there are approximately 19,000 ophthalmologists practicing in the US [34]. Of those, only about 10,000 ophthalmologists perform cataract surgery, with even fewer performing cataract surgery and goniotomy [35]. The surgeon in this report has over 25 years of experience in cataract and glaucoma surgery and in preventing and managing complications to ensure optimal outcomes. We need to train more surgeons to be highly skilled with uncomplicated surgery to ensure excellent outcomes globally.

This study is limited by its retrospective design and absence of a control group. This makes it challenging to infer conclusions of causality between our procedure and the observed outcomes. Though these results are promising and show consistency with those demonstrated in larger clinical trials of other MIGS, utilizing a prospective design with a comparison group as a control arm (e.g., standard cataract surgery alone or other MIGS techniques) in future studies would strengthen the internal validity. Though we did not measure lens thickness in this study, future interventional studies should incorporate this variable to gain a deeper understanding of how lens removal and MIGS can contribute to IOP reduction in different types of glaucoma.

5. Conclusions

Early cataract surgery combined with goniotomy using a Sinskey hook serves as an effective microinvasive surgical alternative, demonstrating reduced intraocular pressure and decreased reliance on ocular hypertensive medications in a cohort primarily composed of Black and Afro-Latino patients with glaucoma, with the outcomes tracked over a 1-year follow-up period. Further research and increased levels of participation from patients of diverse backgrounds are needed to gain a true assessment of the safety and efficacy of glaucoma treatments and interventions in these populations. Longer-term prospective studies that assess the clinical outcomes and economic impact of this combined surgery are necessary to have a better representation of its effects on this chronic, life-long disease.

Author Contributions: Conceptualization, D.L.; methodology, D.L. and I.C.; software, D.L. and I.C.; validation, D.L. and I.C.; formal analysis, D.L. and I.C.; investigation, D.L. and IC.; resources, D.L.; data curation, D.L. and I.C.; writing—original draft preparation, I.C.; writing—review and editing, D.L. and I.C.; visualization, D.L. and I.C.; supervision, D.L.; project administration, D.L. All authors have read and agreed to the published version of the manuscript.

Funding: This research received no external funding.

Institutional Review Board Statement: The study was conducted in accordance with the Declaration of Helsinki. This study, which included human participants, adhered to the ethical standards set by the Icahn School of Medicine Institutional Review Board (IRB), approval code: STUDY-20-00035-CR00, approval date:15 December 2024.

Informed Consent Statement: Informed consent was waived due to the retrospective nature of the study, as approved by the Icahn School of Medicine of Mount Sinai IRB.

Data Availability Statement: The data presented in this study are available upon request from the corresponding author due to the privacy of patient information.

Acknowledgments: The authors thank Louis R. Pasquale and Harriet Lloyd from the Einhorn Clinical Research Center at New York Eye and Ear Infirmary of Mount Sinai for administrative support. Finally, the authors thank the staff at Advance Eye Care of New York for their assistance and support.

Conflicts of Interest: Daniel Laroche has received research support from Nidek and Alcon and is a Speaker for Sight Sciences.

References

1. Ehrlich, J.R.; Burke-Conte, Z.; Wittenborn, J.S.; Saaddine, J.; Omura, J.D.; Friedman, D.S.; Flaxman, A.D.; Rein, D.B. Prevalence of Glaucoma Among US Adults in 2022. *JAMA Ophthalmol.* **2024**, *142*, 1046–1053. [CrossRef] [PubMed]
2. Sommer, A.; Tielsch, J.M.; Katz, J.; Quigley, H.A.; Gottsch, J.D.; Javitt, J.; Singh, K. Relationship between intraocular pressure and primary open angle glaucoma among white and black Americans: The Baltimore Eye Survey. *Arch. Ophthalmol.* **1991**, *109*, 1090–1095. [CrossRef]
3. Heijl, A.; Leske, M.C.; Bengtsson, B.; Hyman, L.; Bengtsson, B.; Hussein, M.; Early Manifest Glaucoma Trial Group. Reduction of intraocular pressure and glaucoma progression: Results from the Early Manifest Glaucoma Trial. *Arch. Ophthalmol.* **2002**, *120*, 1268–1279. [CrossRef] [PubMed]
4. Newman-Casey, P.A.; Niziol, L.M.; Gillespie, B.W.; Janz, N.K.; Lichter, P.R.; Musch, D.C. The Association between Medication Adherence and Visual Field Progression in the Collaborative Initial Glaucoma Treatment Study. *Ophthalmology* **2020**, *127*, 477–483. [CrossRef]
5. Shu, Y.H.; Wu, J.; Luong, T.; Mattox, C.; Fang, E.N.; Lee, B.L.; Jones, J.P.; Campbell, J.; Shih, V.; Zhao, C.; et al. Topical Medication Adherence and Visual Field Progression in Open-angle Glaucoma: Analysis of a Large US Health Care System. *J. Glaucoma* **2021**, *30*, 1047–1055. [CrossRef]
6. Salowe, R.; Salinas, J.; Farbman, N.H.; Mohammed, A.; Warren, J.Z.; Rhodes, A.; Brucker, A.; Regina, M.; Miller-Ellis, E.; Sankar, P.S.; et al. Primary Open-Angle Glaucoma in Individuals of African Descent: A Review of Risk Factors. *J. Clin. Exp. Ophthalmol.* **2015**, *6*, 450. [CrossRef] [PubMed]
7. Racette, L.; Wilson, M.R.; Zangwill, L.M.; Weinreb, R.N.; Sample, P.A. Primary open-angle glaucoma in blacks: A review. *Surv. Ophthalmol.* **2003**, *48*, 295–313. [CrossRef] [PubMed]
8. The Advanced Glaucoma Intervention Study (AGIS): 3. Baseline characteristics of black and white patients. *Ophthalmology* **1998**, *105*, 1137–1145. [CrossRef]
9. Laroche, D.; Capellan, P. The Aging Lens and Glaucoma in persons over 50: Why early cataract surgery/refractive lensectomy and microinvasive trabecular bypass can prevent blindness and cure elevated eye pressure. *J. Natl. Med. Assoc.* **2021**, *113*, 471–473. [CrossRef]
10. Allison, K.; Patel, D.G.; Greene, L. Racial and Ethnic Disparities in Primary Open-Angle Glaucoma Clinical Trials: A Systematic Review and Meta-analysis. *JAMA Netw. Open.* **2021**, *4*, e218348. [CrossRef]
11. Kitayama, K.; Wilson, M.R. Glaucoma in Black Individuals: How Far Have We Come and Where Do We Go From Here? *Am. J. Ophthalmol.* 2023, *Advance online publication*. [CrossRef]
12. Masis, M.; Mineault, P.J.; Phan, E.; Lin, S.C. The role of phacoemulsification in glaucoma therapy: A systematic review and meta-analysis. *Surv. Ophthalmol.* **2018**, *63*, 700–710. [CrossRef] [PubMed]
13. Ling, J.D.; Bell, N.P. Role of Cataract Surgery in the Management of Glaucoma. *Int. Ophthalmol. Clin.* **2018**, *58*, 87–100. [CrossRef] [PubMed]
14. Azuara-Blanco, A.; Burr, J.; Ramsay, C.; Cooper, D.; Foster, P.J.; Friedman, D.S.; Scotland, G.; Javanbakht, M.; Cochrane, C.; Norrie, J.; et al. Effectiveness of early lens extraction for the treatment of primary angle-closure glaucoma (EAGLE): A randomised controlled trial. *Lancet* **2016**, *388*, 1389–1397. [CrossRef]

15. Chen, P.P.; Lin, S.C.; Junk, A.K.; Radhakrishnan, S.; Singh, K.; Chen, T.C. The effect of phacoemulsification on intraocular pressure in glaucoma patients: A report by the American Academy of Ophthalmology. *Ophthalmology* **2015**, *122*, 1294–1307. [CrossRef]
16. Laroche, D.; Oseni, J.; Nkrumah, G.; Ng, C. Clear Lensectomy with Hydrus Stent in Black and Afro-Latino Patients: A 1-Year Retrospective Study. *J. Ophthalmol.* **2022**, *1*, 8011745. [CrossRef] [PubMed]
17. Laroche, D.; Adebayo, A.; Ng, C. Two-Year Retrospective Study of Cataract Surgery and Schlemm Canal Hydrus Microstent in Black and Afro-Latino Patients. *Clin. Ophthalmol.* **2024**, *18*, 2843–2849. [CrossRef] [PubMed]
18. Acuff, K.; Radha Saseendrakumar, B.; Wu, J.H.; Weinreb, R.N.; Baxter, S.L. Racial, Ethnic, and Socioeconomic Disparities in Glaucoma Onset and Severity in a Diverse Nationwide Cohort in the United States. *J. Glaucoma* **2023**, *32*, 792–799. [CrossRef]
19. Laroche, D.; Adebayo, A.; Brown, A.; Ng, C.; Sakkari, S. Early cataract surgery and affordable Sinskey hook goniotomy in Black and Afro-Latino glaucoma patients: A 6-month retrospective study. *Front. Ophthalmol.* **2024**, *4*, 1294651. [CrossRef]
20. Sood, S.; Heilenbach, N.; Sanchez, V.; Glied, S.; Chen, S.; Al-Aswad, L.A. Cost-Effectiveness Analysis of Minimally Invasive Trabecular Meshwork Stents with Phacoemulsification. *Ophthalmol. Glaucoma* **2022**, *5*, 284–296. [CrossRef]
21. Omoto, T.; Fujishiro, T.; Asano-Shimizu, K.; Sugimoto, K.; Sakata, R.; Murata, H.; Asaoka, R.; Honjo, M.; Aihara, M. Comparison of the Short-Term Effectiveness and Safety Profile of Ab Interno Combined Trabeculotomy Using 2 Types of Trabecular Hooks. *Jpn. J. Ophthalmol.* **2020**, *64*, 407–413. [CrossRef]
22. Ahmed, I.I.K.; De Francesco, T.; Rhee, D.; McCabe, C.; Flowers, B.; Gazzard, G.; Samuelson, T.W.; Singh, K.; HORIZON Investigators. Long-Term Outcomes from the HORIZON Randomized Trial for a Schlemm's Canal Microstent in Combination Cataract and Glaucoma Surgery. *Ophthalmology* **2022**, *129*, 742–751. [CrossRef] [PubMed]
23. Vold, S.; Ahmed, I.I.; Craven, E.R.; Mattox, C.; Stamper, R.; Packer, M.; Brown, R.H.; Ianchulev, T.; CyPass Study Group. Two-Year COMPASS Trial Results: Supraciliary Microstenting with Phacoemulsification in Patients with Open-Angle Glaucoma and Cataracts. *Ophthalmology* **2016**, *123*, 2103–2112. [CrossRef]
24. Cantor, L.; Lindfield, D.; Ghinelli, F.; Świder, A.W.; Torelli, F.; Steeds, C.; Dickerson, J.E., Jr.; Nguyen, D.Q. Systematic Literature Review of Clinical, Economic, and Humanistic Outcomes Following Minimally Invasive Glaucoma Surgery or Selective Laser Trabeculoplasty for the Treatment of Open-Angle Glaucoma with or Without Cataract Extraction. *Clin. Ophthalmol.* **2023**, *17*, 85–101. [CrossRef]
25. Falkenberry, S.; Singh, I.P.; Crane, C.J.; Haider, M.A.; Morgan, M.G.; Grenier, C.P.; Brubaker, J.W.; Balasubramani, G.K.; Dorairaj, S. Excisional Goniotomy vs Trabecular Microbypass Stent Implantation: A Prospective Randomized Clinical Trial in Eyes with Mild to Moderate Open-Angle Glaucoma. *J. Cataract. Refract. Surg.* **2020**, *46*, 1165–1171. [CrossRef]
26. Dorairaj, S.K.; Seibold, L.K.; Radcliffe, N.M.; Aref, A.A.; Jimenez-Román, J.; Lazcano-Gomez, G.S.; Darlington, J.K.; Mansouri, K.; Berdahl, J.P. 12-Month Outcomes of Goniotomy Performed Using the Kahook Dual Blade Combined with Cataract Surgery in Eyes with Medically Treated Glaucoma. *Adv. Ther.* **2018**, *35*, 1460–1469. [CrossRef] [PubMed]
27. Sieck, E.G.; Epstein, R.S.; Kennedy, J.B.; SooHoo, J.R.; Pantcheva, M.B.; Patnaik, J.L.; Wagner, B.D.; Lynch, A.M.; Kahook, M.Y.; Seibold, L.K. Outcomes of Kahook Dual Blade Goniotomy with and without Phacoemulsification Cataract Extraction. *Ophthalmol. Glaucoma* **2018**, *1*, 75–81. [CrossRef] [PubMed]
28. Newman-Casey, P.A.; Blachley, T.; Lee, P.P.; Heisler, M.; Farris, K.B.; Stein, J.D. Patterns of Glaucoma Medication Adherence over Four Years of Follow-Up. *Ophthalmology* **2015**, *122*, 2010–2021. [CrossRef]
29. Lee, D.; King, J.; Thomsen, S.; Hirabayashi, M.; An, J. Comparison of Surgical Outcomes Between Excisional Goniotomy Using the Kahook Dual Blade and iStent Trabecular Micro-Bypass Stent in Combination with Phacoemulsification. *Clin. Ophthalmol.* **2019**, *13*, 2097–2102. [CrossRef]
30. Lee, P.P.; Walt, J.G.; Doyle, J.J.; Kotak, S.V.; Evans, S.J.; Budenz, D.L.; Chen, P.P.; Coleman, A.L.; Feldman, R.M.; Jampel, H.D.; et al. A Multicenter, Retrospective Pilot Study of Resource Use and Costs Associated with Severity of Disease in Glaucoma. *Arch. Ophthalmol.* **2006**, *124*, 12–19. [CrossRef]
31. Kyari, F.; Adekoya, B.; Abdull, M.M.; Mohammed, A.S.; Garba, F. The Current Status of Glaucoma and Glaucoma Care in Sub-Saharan Africa. *Asia-Pac. J. Ophthalmol.* **2018**, *7*, 375–386. [CrossRef]
32. Olawoye, O.; Sarimiye, T.; Washaya, J.; Gessesse, G.W.; Balo, K.; Agre, J.; Macheka, B.; Kizor-Akaraiwe, N.; Pons, J.; Ashaye, A.; et al. STAGE Research Group. Patients' Acceptance of Glaucoma Therapy in Sub-Saharan Africa. *J. Glaucoma* **2024**, *33*, 951–956. [CrossRef] [PubMed]
33. Nganga Ngabou, C.G.F.; Makita, C.; Ndalla, S.S.; Nkokolo, F.; Madzou, M. Baisse de la Pression Intraoculaire Après Chirurgie Manuelle de la Cataracte par Petite Incision [Intraocular Pressure Decrease After Manual Small Incision Cataract Surgery]. *J. Fr. Ophtalmol.* **2017**, *40*, 397–402. [CrossRef] [PubMed]

34. Association of American Medical Colleges. U.S. Physician Workforce Data Dashboard [Internet]. 2023. Available online: https://www.aamc.org/data-reports/report/us-physician-workforce-data-dashboard (accessed on 15 February 2025).
35. Bhatnagar, A.; Skrehot, H.; Ahmed, M. County Variation in Cataract Surgery Access in the United States. *Investig. Ophthalmol. Vis. Sci.* **2023**, *64*, OD52.

Journal of
Clinical Medicine

Article

Comparison of Efficacy and Ocular Surface Assessment Between Preserved and Preservative-Free Brimonidine/Timolol Fixed-Combination Eye Drops in Glaucoma Patients: A Parallel-Grouped, Randomized Trial

Myungjin Kim [1], Chang-Kyu Lee [2], Jonghoon Shin [3,4,5], Doah Kim [1] and Seungsoo Rho [1,*]

1 Department of Ophthalmology, CHA Bundang Medical Center, CHA University, Seongnam 13496, Republic of Korea; brandmjeyes@gmail.com (M.K.); inhamed93216006@gmail.com (D.K.)
2 Department of Ophthalmology, Ulsan University Hospital, University of Ulsan College of Medicine, Ulsan 44033, Republic of Korea; coolleo@uuh.ulsan.kr
3 Department of Ophthalmology, Pusan National University Yangsan Hospital, Pusan National University School of Medicine, Yangsan 50612, Republic of Korea; jjonggal@naver.com
4 Research Institute for Convergence of Biomedical Science and Technology, Pusan National University Yangsan Hospital, Yangsan 50612, Republic of Korea
5 PNU Busan Eye Clinic, Busan 46241, Republic of Korea
* Correspondence: harryrho@gmail.com; Tel.: +82-31-780-5330

Abstract: The objectives of the study were to compare the efficacy and safety using ocular surface assessment between preserved and preservative-free brimonidine/timolol fixed-combination eye drops in glaucoma or ocular hypertension patients. **Methods**: This study was designed as a prospective, multicenter (three institutions), investigator-masked, parallel-grouped randomized clinical trial. The primary outcomes were corneal and conjunctival staining score, ocular surface disease index (OSDI) score, drug tolerance, and adherence rates at 12-week visits. The secondary outcomes were corneal and conjunctival staining score, OSDI score at 4-week visits and intraocular pressure (IOP), tear-film breakup time (TBUT), and bulbar/limbal hyperemia score at the 4- and 12-week visits. For safety assessment, best-corrected visual acuity (BCVA), systolic blood pressure (SBP), diastolic blood pressure (DBP), heart rate (HR), and physical examination at 4 and 12 weeks and adverse events during the whole study period were analyzed. **Results**: Overall, 59 patients were enrolled and randomized into each group (29 preserved and 30 preservative-free). At the endpoint, 5 patients in the preserved group and 2 patients in the preservative-free group dropped out, leaving 24 and 28 patients in the preserved and preservative-free groups, respectively. Baseline characteristics showed no significant difference between the groups including age and sex. At the 12-week visit, intra-group change of OSDI scores did not change significantly compared to the baseline scores in both preserved and preservative-free groups (p = 0.791, 0.478, respectively). On the contrary, the corneal staining score and the conjunctival staining score showed a significant increase compared to the baseline score in the preserved group (p = 0.015, 0.009, respectively). Regarding drug satisfaction, higher proportions of patients in the preservative-free group reported convenience of installation (p = 0.002). Also, stinging and burning sensations in drug tolerance showed better results in the preservative-free group with a significant difference (p = 0.011). Safety assessment regarding systemic side effects such as SBP, DBP, and HR showed similar results between the preserved and preservative-free groups (p = 0.711, 0.232, 0.666, respectively). **Conclusions**: Preservative-free brimonidine/timolol showed comparable efficacy and safety, better corneal and conjunctival staining score with convenience of installation, and lower stinging and burning sensation. It is expected to be a proper treatment option for patients with glaucoma or ocular hypertension.

Keywords: preservative-free; brimonidine/timolol; glaucoma; ocular hypertension; efficacy; safety; corneal staining score; conjunctival staining score; ocular surface disease index; drug tolerance; adherence

1. Introduction

Medication adherence is crucial for achieving optimal treatment outcomes regardless of a wide range of diseases. By identifying and addressing the drivers and barriers to adherence, physicians can better support their patients in adhering to their medication regimens, ultimately leading to improved treatment outcomes. However, a review spanning three decades found that between 30% and 50% of patients exhibit poor compliance with their prescribed treatments, regardless of disease type, prognosis, or care setting [1]. Glaucoma, which is characterized by chronic progressive damage to the optic nerve, is often asymptomatic until the advanced stage, making it more prone to poor patient adherence and persistence [2–5].

Previous studies have shown that factors such as younger age, male, poor general health status, and psychiatric conditions like depression negatively impact adherence to glaucoma medications [6–8]. In addition to these patient factors, the adherence rate may be dependent on the medication itself. As eyedrops contain not only active pharmaceutical ingredients but also excipients (non-active pharmaceutical ingredients) and preservatives, it is essential to thoroughly consider the potential impact of all these components when assessing their influence on adherence.

When administering eyedrops, several routes of absorption are possible and excessive amounts of active ingredients may cause unwanted systemic side effects. For example, brimonidine can lead to systemic adverse reactions, including dry mouth, dizziness, fatigue, and drowsiness, especially in predisposed bradycardic patients [9,10]. Eye drops with timolol also can have a strong and prolonged systemic effect such as decreased heart rate or cardiac output, and syncope especially in older age groups [10–12].

In addition to systemic effects, preservatives in the eye drops have been demonstrated to increase the patients' discomfort associated with the therapy, contributing to the development of ocular surface disease (OSD) [13]. Benzalkonium chloride (BAK), a common preservative in ophthalmic solutions, is effective at preventing bacterial and fungal growth [14]. However, this cytotoxic property can also harm ocular surface cells, and studies indicate a correlation between the number of BAK-preserved drops used and the occurrence of adverse ocular surface signs and symptoms [15–20]. This association is further supported by observed improvements in ocular surface signs and symptoms followed by a discontinuation of the preserved drops and switch to preservative-free drops [18,21]. The occurrence of OSD in glaucoma patients is a considerable problem as it could be associated with reduced patients' adherence to glaucoma eyedrop which leads to treatment failure [15–17,21–24]. Thus, the use of preservative-free eye drops becomes more popular, as they are likely to reduce or eliminate ocular side effects of preservatives.

Recently, a preservative-free brimonidine/timolol fixed-combination eyedrop has been developed in South Korea. The main purpose of this study was to prospectively compare the efficacy and safety of preservative-free brimonidine/timolol (Bridin plus®, Hanlim Pharm, Seoul, Republic of Korea) to preserved brimonidine/timolol (Combigan™, Allergan Inc., Irvine, CA, USA) in aspects of ocular surface assessment and adherence rates in patients with open-angle glaucoma or ocular hypertension. This study is a serial investigation following our prior research, which prospectively compared preserved and preservative-free latanoprost, and preserved and preservative-free brimonidine tartrate [25,26]. Moreover, to evaluate the potential benefits of preservative-free brimonidine/timolol, systemic parameters, questionnaire-based patient satisfaction, and drug tolerance scores were analyzed.

2. Materials and Methods

2.1. Study Design and Subject Enrollment

This prospective, multicenter (three institutions), investigator-masked, parallel-grouped randomized clinical trial aimed to assess the efficacy and safety of preserved and preservative-free brimonidine/timolol in patients with open-angle glaucoma or ocular hypertension. The study was approved by the institutional review boards of CHA Bundang Medical Center, Pusan National University Yangsan Hospital, and Ulsan University Hospital, adhered to the tenets of the Declaration of Helsinki, and was registered on clinicaltrials.gov on 8 October 2021 (NCT06078592). All subjects were enrolled from October 2021 to December 2022.

Glaucomatous changes in the eye were confirmed by consistent glaucomatous visual field defects that corresponded with characteristic optic disc and retinal nerve fiber layer abnormalities, as assessed by glaucoma specialists [27,28]. Each participant underwent a comprehensive ophthalmologic examination, which included best-corrected visual acuity (BCVA) measured using Snellen chart [29], intraocular pressure (IOP) assessment via Goldmann applanation tonometry by masked examiners in each institution [30,31], central corneal thickness (CCT) [30,32], gonioscopy [33,34], visual field test with a Humphrey Field Analyzer (Carl Zeiss Meditec, Dublin, CA, USA) [35], fundus photography (Carl Zeiss Meditec, Dublin, CA, USA) [36], red-free photography (Carl Zeiss Meditec, Dublin, CA, USA) [36], and spectral-domain optical coherence tomography (Carl Zeiss Meditec, Dublin, CA, USA) [37–39]. Additionally, baseline physical characteristics such as height and weight, were recorded using a standardized stadiometer and digital scale, with participants wearing light clothing and no shoes.

To be included in the study, patients needed to have an IOP between 15 and 40 mmHg in at least one eye during the screening visit, following the appropriate washout period. Exclusion criteria included BCVA worse than Snellen 20/80 (decimal 0.25), CCT outside the range of 470 to 591 μm, and any ocular condition (e.g., ischemic optic neuropathy, proliferative diabetic retinopathy, age-related macular degeneration) that could significantly affect visual field results. Patients with active ocular inflammatory conditions, a history of lacrimal punctal occlusion procedures within the past three months, or a need for eyedrops containing hyaluronic acid, cyclosporine, or diquafosol for severe dry eye disease were also excluded. Also, pregnant or currently nursing individuals were not eligible for participation.

All participants receiving IOP-lowering treatment underwent a washout period of four weeks, except for those using cholinergic eye drops and carbonic anhydrase inhibitors, who had a shorter washout period of five days. After the washout phase, they were randomly assigned to one of two groups: one receiving multi-dose preserved brimonidine/timolol (Combigan™, Allergan Inc., Irvine, CA, USA) and the other receiving unit-dose preservative-free brimonidine/timolol (Bridin plus®, Hanlim Pharm, Seoul, Republic of Korea).

Randomization was conducted centrally and automatically using an interactive web-based randomization system (IWRS, TnW software Ltd., Seoul, Republic of Korea), which operated 24/7 throughout the study period. All patient data and study variables were recorded in a web-based electronic case report form (ver 1.0, http://www.ecrf.kr (accessed on 31 December 2022), TnW software Ltd., Seoul, Republic of Korea). To ensure masking, both treatment groups received their respective study medications in identical external packaging. While patients were aware of their assigned treatment, investigators remained blinded to the treatment allocation throughout the study period. The patients were instructed to instill either preserved or preservative-free brimonidine/timolol twice daily from day 0 and to visit the clinic at 4 and 12 weeks (Figure 1A). At both 4- and 12-week visits, the patients underwent follow-up measurements at 10 AM ± 1 h and instilled the eyedrops thereafter.

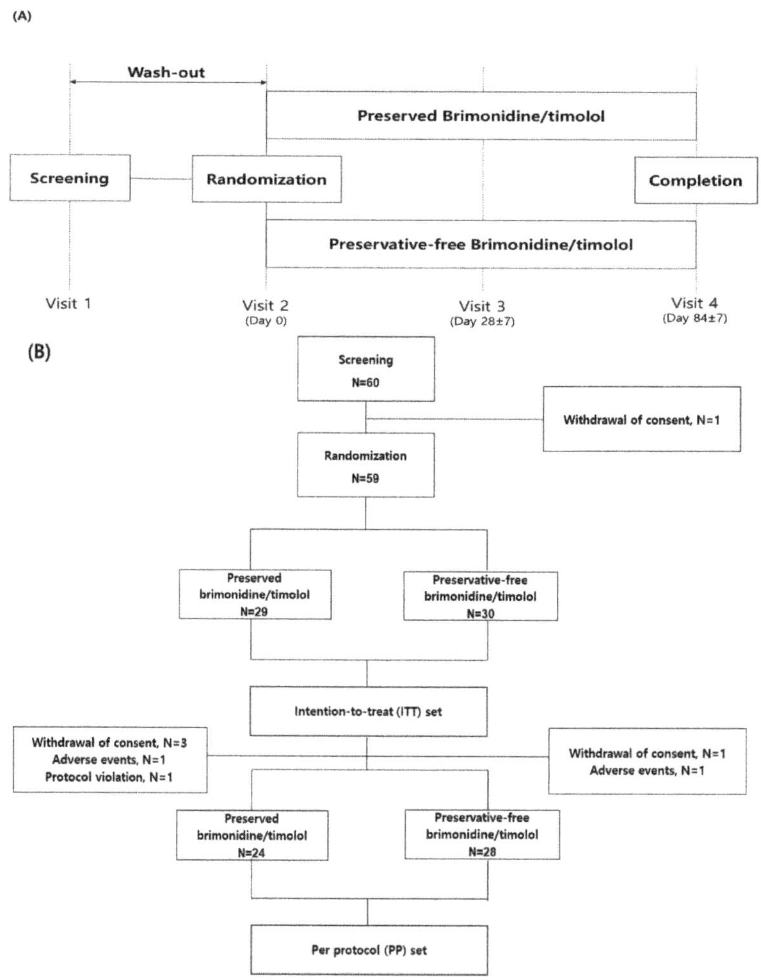

Figure 1. Flow chart of the study: (**A**) follow-up schedule; (**B**) subjects' enrollment.

2.2. Outcome Measurements

The investigators performed evaluations at both the 4-week and 12-week visits (at 10 AM ± 1 h), ensuring consistency in capturing time-sensitive signs and symptoms. The primary endpoints were the difference in the corneal staining grade assessed by the Oxford grading system (0–5) and conjunctival staining score assessed by the National Eye Institute scale (0–3) [40,41] with FLUO 900 fluorescein strip (Haag-Streit, Köniz, Switzerland) staining under the slit lamp examination using a cobalt blue light. The ocular surface disease index (OSDI) score [42], drug tolerance, and adherence rates at 12-week visits were obtained. The drug tolerance data were acquired using a questionnaire sheet to evaluate the frequency and severity of the symptoms associated with using eye drops, including stinging/burning, sticky sensation, itching, blurring, sandiness/grittiness, dryness, light sensitivity, and pain/soreness. The level of each symptom was graded as 0 (none) to 3 (severe, immensely interfering with the subject's daily life), and the duration of each symptom as 0 (prompt: <5 min) or 1 (continuous: ≥5 min). Adherence rates (0–100%) were assessed at 4 and 12 weeks using a self-report sheet [25,26].

The secondary efficacy endpoints were corneal and conjunctival staining score, and OSDI score at 4-week visits and IOP measured by Goldmann applanation, tear break-up time (TBUT) with FLUO 900 fluorescein strip staining under the slit lamp examination using a cobalt blue light, and bulbar and limbal hyperemia score assessed by Efron grading scale (0–4) [43] at the 4- and 12–week visits. For safety assessment, BCVA, systolic blood pressure (SBP), diastolic blood pressure (DBP), heart rate (HR) at 4 and 12 weeks, and adverse events (AEs) during the whole study period were analyzed.

2.3. Statistical Analysis

This study aimed to evaluate the superiority of preservative-free brimonidine/timolol over preserved brimonidine/timolol in terms of ocular surface. Superiority was concluded if the difference in the hyperemia score was 0.82 or more according to a study that evaluated the difference in eye redness before and after switching the subjects using preserved and preservative-free eyedrops [25,26,44,45]. Assuming a dropout rate of 25% and a standard deviation of 1.0 for the hyperemia score, a total of 60 patients (30 in each group) were required to achieve 90% power for the superiority calculation, resulting in a minimal sample size of 21 per group after accounting for dropouts [25,26,44,45]. To maximize the accuracy of the assessment among all investigators, a blinded person created a validation image set of conjunctival hyperemia, which was used to check the agreement between each investigator [25,26,44,45].

Baseline characteristics were compared between the preserved and preservative-free groups using independent t-tests or Wilcoxon rank-sum tests for continuous variables and chi-square or Fisher's exact tests for categorical variables. Prior to selecting statistical tests, the normality of data distributions was assessed using the Shapiro–Wilk test. Variables that followed a normal distribution were analyzed using parametric tests, while non-parametric methods were used for non-normally distributed data. Inter-group comparisons of continuous outcome measurements at 4- and 12-week visits were performed using analysis of covariance (ANCOVA) after adjusting baseline values and covariates, if needed. Intra-group comparisons of serial measurements compared to baseline data were performed using paired t-test or Wilcoxon signed-rank tests. Assessments were performed using intention-to-treat (ITT) and per-protocol (PP) sets. Only patients who did not violate the protocol with an adherence rate of more than 80% were included in the PP set. Statistical analyses were performed using the Statistical Package for the Social Sciences for Windows (version 18.0; IBM Corp., Armonk, NY, USA), and statistical significance was set at $p < 0.05$.

3. Results

Overall, 59 patients were randomized into each group (29 preserved and 30 preservative-free group) which comprised an ITT set. During the study, five patients (three withdrawal of consent, one adverse event, one protocol violation) were excluded from the preserved group and two patients (one withdrawal of consent, one adverse event) from the preservative-free group. Consequently, 24 and 28 patients were included in the PP set of preserved and preservative-free groups, respectively (Figure 1B). There were no significant differences in the demographic and baseline features including age and sex, between the groups, minimizing potential confounding effects on variables such as BCVA, SBP, DBP, and HR (Table 1).

Table 1. Demographic and baseline characteristics between the preserved and preservative-free brimonidine/timolol groups (ITT set). *SBP*, systolic blood pressure; *DBP*, diastolic blood pressure; *HR*, heart rate; *BCVA*, best-corrected visual acuity; *IOP*, intraocular pressure; *CCT*, central corneal thickness; *OSDI*, ocular surface disease index.

	Preserved (n = 29)	Preservative-Free (n = 30)	p
Age, years	59.21 ± 11.47	57.27 ± 12.42	0.480
Male, n (%)	18 (62.1)	18 (60.0)	0.871
Duration of disease, years	0.45 ± 2.17	1.19 ± 3.52	0.834
Height, cm	166.07 ± 8.21	165.12 ± 7.33	0.640
Weight, kg	67.43 ± 10.89	67.23 ± 10.34	0.945
SBP, mmHg	129.21 ± 12.68	131.83 ± 14.01	0.454
DBP, mmHg	76.72 ± 9.34	78.10 ± 10.51	0.597
HR, beat per minute	75.69 ± 9.01	78.57 ± 9.08	0.249
BCVA (decimal)	0.88 ± 0.26	0.92 ± 0.22	0.512
IOP, mmHg	19.21 ± 2.84	18.71 ± 3.31	0.309
CCT, μm	546.76 ± 34.20	544.03 ± 27.24	0.499
Bulbar hyperemia	1.11 ± 0.69	0.83 ± 0.71	0.136
Limbal hyperemia	0.86 ± 0.71	0.79 ± 0.68	0.746
Corneal staining score	0.57 ± 0.69	0.79 ± 0.68	0.192
Conjunctival staining score	0.68 ± 0.62	0.90 ± 0.61	0.152
Tear film break up time	7.50 ± 6.26	7.69 ± 6.36	0.924
OSDI score	7.86 ± 6.41	7.37 ± 6.10	0.789

3.1. Primary Outcomes

The corneal and conjunctival staining scores, OSDI scores, drug tolerance, and patient satisfaction at 12-week visits were compared between the groups (Table 2). Although the corneal and conjunctival staining scores and OSDI scores did not differ significantly between the preserved and preservative-free groups at 12-week visits (Table 2), comparing intra-group changes of the corneal and conjunctival staining scores at 12-week visits from the baseline score for each group, preserved group showed increased corneal score in ITT set and increased conjunctival score in both the ITT and PP set, which means an increased ocular surface defect of cornea and conjunctiva in the preserved brimonidine/timolol group (Figures 2 and 3).

Regarding drug tolerance, a stinging/burning sensation was more often associated with the preserved group in both ITT and PP sets with statistical significance ($p = 0.011$, 0.010, respectively; Table 2). Pain/soreness sensation was also higher in the preserved group in the PP set with statistical significance ($p = 0.033$; Table 2). In the patient satisfaction score, the preservative-free group reported that the unit-dose container was easier for installation in both ITT and PP set with statistical significance ($p = 0.004$, 0.002, respectively; Table 2), and easier for storage in the PP set with statistical significance ($p = 0.030$; Table 2).

Table 2. Primary outcome measurements at 12-week visit. *OSDI* ocular surface disease index. [a] Statistical analyses were conducted using ANCOVA after adjusting baseline data. [b] Statistical analyses were conducted using independent *t*-test or Wilcoxon's rank sum test. Significant values with $p < 0.05$ are indicated in bold.

	Intention-to-Treat Set			Per-Protocol Set		
	Preserved (n = 29)	Preservative-Free (n = 30)	*p*	Preserved (n = 24)	Preservative-Free (n = 28)	*p*
Corneal staining score (V4)	1.08 ± 0.15	0.75 ± 0.15	0.125 [a]	0.91 ± 0.16	0.81 ± 0.14	0.630 [a]
Corneal staining score difference from baseline (V4-baseline)	0.46 ± 0.88	0.00 ± 0.89	0.060	0.33 ± 0.80	0.07 ± 0.87	0.310 [b]
Conjunctival staining score (V4)	1.02 ± 0.09	0.85 ± 0.09	0.211 [a]	1.00 ± 0.11	0.84 ± 0.10	0.325 [a]
Conjunctival staining score difference from baseline (V4-baseline)	0.28 ± 0.53	0.00 ± 0.62	0.073	0.31 ± 0.57	−0.01 ± 0.64	0.084 [b]
OSDI score (V4)	7.65 ± 1.36	6.27 ± 1.34	0.473 [a]	9.49 ± 1.62	6.36 ± 1.43	0.153 [a]
OSDI score difference from baseline (V4-baseline)	0.11 ± 7.92	−1.38 ± 8.02	0.835	1.76 ± 8.09	−1.11 ± 8.02	0.423 [b]
Drug tolerance score						
Stinging/burning	0.82 ± 0.67	0.38 ± 0.49	**0.011**	0.86 ± 0.65	0.37 ± 0.49	**0.010** [b]
Sticky	0.29 ± 0.53	0.10 ± 0.41	0.076	0.29 ± 0.46	0.11 ± 0.42	0.070 [b]
Itching	0.29 ± 0.53	0.28 ± 0.65	0.727	0.29 ± 0.56	0.30 ± 0.67	0.910 [b]
Blurred vision	0.54 ± 0.64	0.38 ± 0.56	0.341	0.62 ± 0.67	0.37 ± 0.56	0.173 [b]
Sandiness/grittiness	0.36 ± 0.56	0.17 ± 0.38	0.182	0.38 ± 0.50	0.19 ± 0.40	0.138 [b]
Dryness	0.43 ± 0.74	0.28 ± 0.45	0.603	0.48 ± 0.75	0.30 ± 0.47	0.486 [b]
Light sensitivity	0.17 ± 0.47	0.43 ± 0.69	0.100	0.19 ± 0.48	0.52 ± 0.75	0.064 [b]
Pain/soreness	0.36 ± 0.49	0.17 ± 0.38	0.120	0.43 ± 0.51	0.15 ± 0.36	**0.033** [b]
Patient satisfaction score						
Easy to open	1.61 ± 0.74	1.31 ± 0.54	0.109	1.71 ± 0.78	1.33 ± 0.55	0.075 [b]
Easy for installation	1.89 ± 0.74	1.38 ± 0.68	**0.004**	2.05 ± 0.74	1.41 ± 0.69	**0.002** [b]
Easy for storage	1.61 ± 0.69	1.38 ± 0.62	0.163	1.81 ± 0.68	1.41 ± 0.64	**0.030** [b]
Easy for drug management	1.39 ± 0.74	1.17 ± 0.47	0.251	1.52 ± 0.81	1.19 ± 0.48	0.110 [b]

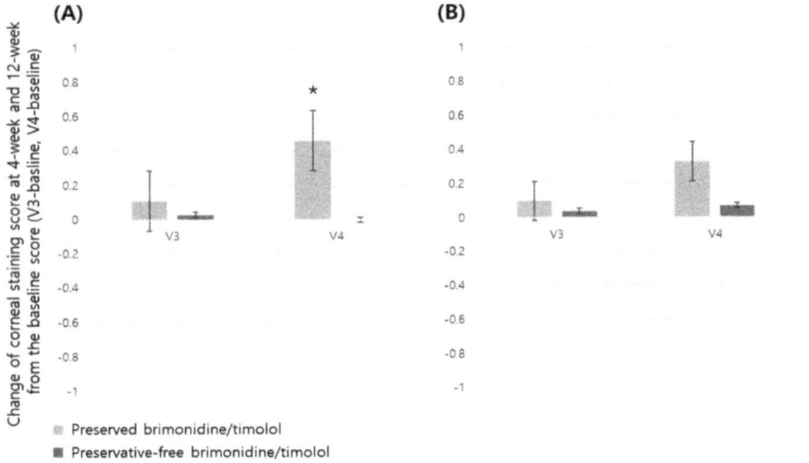

Figure 2. Intra-group change of corneal staining scores in preserved and preservative-free brimonidine/timolol groups at 4-week (V3) and 12-week (V4) visits from the baseline score. (* represents

statistical significance by paired *t*-test). ITT, intention-to-treat set; PP, per-protocol set. (**A**) ITT, intention-to-treat set; (**B**) PP, per-protocol set.

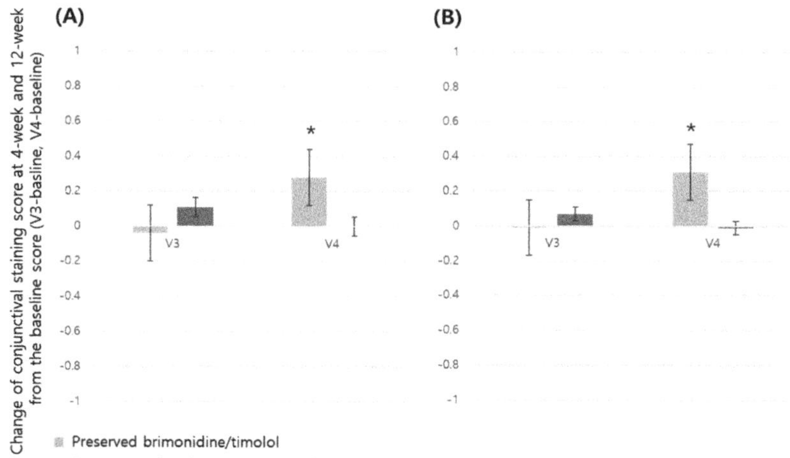

Figure 3. Intra-group change of conjunctival staining score in preserved and preservative-free brimonidine/timolol groups at 4-week (V3) and 12-week (V4) visits from the baseline score (* represents statistical significance by paired *t*-test). ITT, intention-to-treat set; PP, per-protocol set. (**A**) ITT, intention-to-treat set; (**B**) PP, per-protocol set.

Adherence rates differed with statistical significance between the groups (Figure 4). At 4-week visits, the preserved group reported an adherence rate of 95.42%, while the preservative-free group reported 98.86% ($p = 0.003$). At 12-week visits, the adherence rate of the preserved group decreased to 90.44%, while the preservative-free group increased to 98.86% ($p = 0.036$).

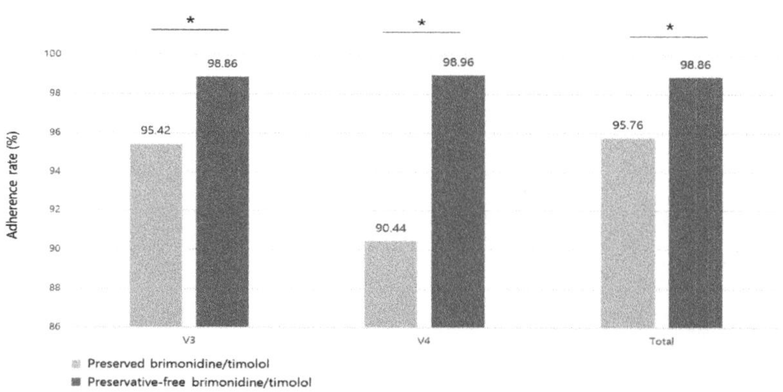

Figure 4. Adherence rate (%) between preserved and preservative-free brimonidine/timolol groups. (* represents statistical significance by independent *t*-test).

3.2. Secondary Outcomes

There were no statistically significant differences between the groups in corneal and conjunctival staining score and OSDI score at 4-week visits. Also, the TBUT score and bulbar/limbal hyperemic score did not differ significantly between the groups at 4-week and 12-week (Table 3) visits. However, intra-group differences of the OSDI score were observed in the preservative-free group at 4-week visits in the ITT set, and in both preserved and preservative-free groups at 4-week visits in the PP set (Figure 5). In addition, although both groups showed decreased OSDI scores compared with the baseline at 4-week visits, the OSDI score change showed a different tendency at 12-week visits in both groups. The preserved group showed increased OSDI scores compared with the baseline at 12-week visits, while the preservative-free group showed consistently decreased OSDI scores (Figure 5). Other variables including bulbar and limbal hyperemic score and IOP at 4 and 12 weeks showed no statistically significant differences between the groups. Both groups showed significantly lower IOPs at both 4 and 12 weeks compared to those at baseline, with no significant differences between the groups throughout the study period.

Table 3. Secondary outcome measurements at 4-week visits (V3) and 12-week visits (V4). *OSDI*, ocular surface disease index; *TBUT*, tear-film break up time; *IOP*, intraocular pressure. [a] Statistical analyses were conducted using ANCOVA after adjusting baseline data. [b] Statistical analyses were conducted using independent *t*-test or Wilcoxon's rank sum test.

	Intention-to-Treat Set			**Per-Protocol Set**		
	Preserved (n = 29)	**Preservative-Free (n = 30)**	*p*	**Preserved (n = 24)**	**Preservative-Free (n = 28)**	*p*
Corneal staining score (V3)	0.72 ± 0.13	0.79 ± 0.13	0.702	0.66 ± 0.16	0.78 ± 0.14	0.560 [a]
Corneal staining score difference from baseline (V3-baseline)	0.11 ± 0.83	0.03 ± 0.78	0.619	0.10 ± 0.94	0.04 ± 0.81	0.722 [b]
Conjunctival staining score (V3)	0.71 ± 0.12	0.95 ± 0.12	0.162	0.69 ± 0.14	0.91 ± 0.13	0.264 [a]
Conjunctival staining score difference from baseline (V3-baseline)	−0.04 ± 0.57	0.11 ± 0.77	0.735	−0.01 ± 0.60	0.07 ± 0.76	0.478 [b]
OSDI score (V3)	5.72 ± 0.82	4.52 ± 0.80	0.298	5.81 ± 0.97	4.26 ± 0.85	0.236 [a]
OSDI score difference from baseline (V3-baseline)	−1.82 ± 4.36	−3.14 ± 6.89	0.195	−1.95 ± 4.01	−3.19 ± 7.11	0.452 [b]
TBUT (V3), sec	6.34 ± 0.44	6.55 ± 0.43	0.728	6.24 ± 0.53	6.52 ± 0.47	0.699 [a]
TBUT difference from baseline (V3-baseline)	−0.16 ± 2.57	0.22 ± 2.62	0.892	−0.33 ± 2.90	0.09 ± 2.61	0.604 [b]
TBUT (V4), sec	6.43 ± 0.46	6.69 ± 0.46	0.689	6.54 ± 0.57	6.75 ± 0.51	0.781 [a]
TBUT difference from baseline (V4-baseline)	−0.08 ± 3.05	0.36 ± 2.38	0.550	−0.03 ± 3.30	0.31 ± 2.45	0.683 [b]
Hyperemic score						
Bulbar (V3)	0.55 ± 0.10	0.64 ± 0.10	0.510	0.38 ± 0.11	0.63 ± 0.10	0.101 [a]
Bulbar hyperemic score difference from baseline (V3-baseline)	−0.50 ± 0.69	−0.24 ± 0.64	0.281	−0.67 ± 0.76	−0.26 ± 0.66	0.094 [b]
Bulbar (V4)	0.70 ± 0.10	0.64 ± 0.10	0.659	0.62 ± 0.12	0.63 ± 0.10	0.982 [a]
Bulbar hyperemic score difference from baseline (V4-baseline)	−0.36 ± 0.68	−0.24 ± 0.69	0.774	−0.43 ± 0.75	−0.26 ± 0.71	0.632 [b]
Limbal (V3)	0.56 ± 0.11	0.60 ± 0.11	0.818	0.38 ± 0.13	0.59 ± 0.11	0.221 [a]
Limbal hyperemic score difference from baseline (V3-baseline)	−0.29 ± 0.66	−0.21 ± 0.82	0.956	−0.43 ± 0.68	−0.22 ± 0.85	0.556 [b]
Limbal (V4)	0.81 ± 0.10	0.70 ± 0.10	0.467	0.76 ± 0.13	0.70 ± 0.11	0.721 [a]
Limbal hyperemic score difference from baseline (V4-baseline)	−0.04 ± 0.51	−0.10 ± 0.82	0.507	−0.05 ± 0.59	−0.11 ± 0.80	0.593 [b]

Table 3. *Cont.*

	Intention-to-Treat Set			Per-Protocol Set		
	Preserved (n = 29)	**Preservative-Free (n = 30)**	p	**Preserved (n = 24)**	**Preservative-Free (n = 28)**	p
IOP (V3), mmHg	13.89 ± 0.43	13.32 ± 0.42	0.348	13.16 ± 0.38	13.19 ± 0.33	0.949 [a]
IOP difference from baseline (V3-baseline)	−5.20 ± 2.92	−5.52 ± 2.52	0.785	−6.24 ± 2.19	−5.78 ± 2.35	0.186 [b]
IOP (V4), mmHg	13.71 ± 2.80	12.34 ± 2.45	0.054	13.27 ± 0.48	12.57 ± 0.42	0.280 [a]
IOP difference from baseline (V4-baseline)	−5.50 ± 2.94	−6.36 ± 2.78	0.260	−6.14 ± 2.51	−6.39 ± 2.83	0.755 [b]

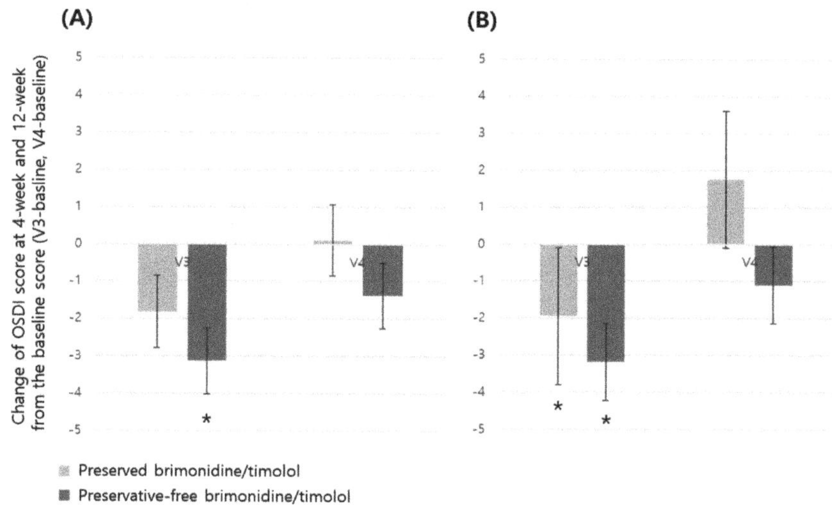

Figure 5. Intra-group change of OSDI score in preserved and preservative-free brimonidine/timolol groups at 4-week (V3) and 12-week (V4) visits from the baseline score. (* represents statistical significance by paired *t*-test). (**A**) ITT, intention-to-treat set; (**B**) PP, per-protocol set.

3.3. Safety Assessments

The BCVA, SBP, DBP, and HR did not differ between the groups throughout the study period, with all variables in the normal range (Table 4). The total incidence of AEs was 25.42% (15/59 patients, 16 cases), which was 24.14% (7/29 patients, 8 cases) in the preserved group and 26.67% (8/30 patients, 8 cases) in the preservative-free group. The AEs that caused the drop-out in the study were palpitations in the preserved group and dizziness in the preservative-free group. However, severe AEs were not reported, and all participants recovered to a normal state after discontinuing the eyedrops.

Table 4. Safety assessment at 4- and 12-week visits using per-protocol set. *BCVA*, best-corrected visual acuity; *SBP*, systolic blood pressure; *DBP*, diastolic blood pressure; *HR*, heart rate. Comparative analyses were performed using ANCOVA after adjusting age, gender, and baseline data, except for BCVA. For BCVA, the Wilcoxon rank-sum test was used.

	4-Week Visit			12-Week Visit		
	Preserved (n = 29)	**Preservative-Free (n = 30)**	p	**Preserved (n = 24)**	**Preservative-Free (n = 28)**	p
BCVA (decimal)	0.90 ± 0.24	0.94 ± 0.25	0.438	0.88 ± 0.24	0.96 ± 0.24	0.145
SBP, mmHg	127.58 ± 9.23	128.39 ± 13.58	0.806	126.18 ± 11.25	128.00 ± 8.02	0.313

Table 4. *Cont.*

	4-Week Visit			12-Week Visit		
	Preserved (n = 29)	Preservative-Free (n = 30)	p	Preserved (n = 24)	Preservative-Free (n = 28)	p
SBP-baseline, mmHg	−1.50 ± 10.88	−2.89 ± 14.04	0.6947	−2.71 ± 11.26	−3.90 ± 12.60	0.7105
DBP, mmHg	76.72 ± 9.34	78.10 ± 10.51	0.598	71.46 ± 6.06	72.34 ± 5.30	0.249
DBP-baseline, mmHg	1.75 ± 9.52	−1.18 ± 9.71	0.2792	1.46 ± 10.96	−1.83 ± 9.59	0.2322
HR, bpm	73.29 ± 7.84	72.07 ± 9.25	0.406	72.34 ± 5.30	71.46 ± 6.06	0.453

4. Discussion

Ocular surface can be affected not only by preservatives like BAK, but also by active pharmaceutical ingredients or other excipients with which BAK is combined. Several in vitro and ex vivo studies have shown that BAK alone, at concentrations commonly found in commercial formulation, and BAK combined with timolol, have more deleterious effects on conjunctival cells compared to BAK used with prostaglandin analogues [46–49]. Similarly, the fact that conjunctiva staining score showed differences between the groups at 4 weeks in our study implies that the active pharmaceutical ingredient should also be under consideration for the cause of OSD. Sherwood et al. [50] demonstrated that in the 12-month clinical trial, the most frequent treatment-related AEs by brimonidine/timolol recipients (n = 385) were conjunctival hyperemia (14.5%), followed by ocular stinging (6.2%), eye pruritus (5.5%), and allergic conjunctivitis (5.2%). Interestingly, ocular stinging was more frequent with brimonidine/timolol therapy than with brimonidine alone ($p = 0.03$), though other adverse events were less common with brimonidine/timolol ($p < 0.02$). These results support the fact that the impact on the ocular surface or ocular side effects can vary depending on the composition of active ingredients as well. On the contrary, our results showed that both bulbar and limbal hyperemic scores rather decreased at 12 weeks compared to baseline scores in both preserved and preservative-free brimonidine/timolol groups, although they did not show statistical differences. The impact of brimonidine/timolol on hyperemia seems to manifest between 3-month and 12-month intervals, highlighting the need for increased attention to conjunctival hyperemia during this period which may be due to allergic reaction. We also evaluated stinging/burning sensation to assess drug tolerance. There were statistically significant differences in the stinging/burning sensation between the preserved and preservative-free groups in both ITT and PP sets. Thus, starting with preservative-free brimonidine/timolol could be beneficial to improve ocular comfort and tolerance from the outset, avoiding potential issues related to hyperemia and ocular discomfort. Also, switching from preserved brimonidine/timolol to preservative-free brimonidine/timolol would be another treatment option for patients experiencing ocular a stinging sensation.

Even with topical administration, brimonidine and timolol can enter systemic circulation, potentially causing cardiovascular (brimonidine, timolol) and pulmonary (timolol) effects [51–54]. Stewart et al. [54], reported that the use of concomitant timolol maleate and brimonidine, given as separate agents, was related with ventricular premature contractions during exercise, and atrial premature contractions during recovery in treatment groups. On the contrary, in our study in which brimonidine and timolol were given in a fixed-combination formula, there were no significant systemic AEs in the safety assessment. The components used in formulating fixed combinations of brimonidine and timolol appear to possess the potential to mitigate these cardiovascular and pulmonary effects associated with each individual use of brimonidine or timolol. Meanwhile, our previous study [26] reported lower SBP and DBP at 4 and 12 weeks compared to baseline measures when using preserved brimonidine, but not in the preservative-free brimonidine group. The important factor could be the extent of individual drug consumption. Since bottle-type dispensers are not transparent, patients may have inadvertently instilled multiple drops at one session, resulting in overconsumption. In contrast, no such association was identified for unit-dose pipettes [55]. Furthermore, the difference in total amount of brimonidine derived from the different frequency of use and the concentration would have influenced the results. In our previous study [26], the brimonidine was required to be instilled three times a day, whereas in the current study, brimonidine/timolol was required to be instilled twice daily. Brimonidin (Alphagan P®, Allergan Inc., Irvine, CA, USA) is typically prescribed as 0.15% administered three times daily, totaling 0.45% per day, whereas brimonidine/timolol (Combigan™, Allergan Inc., Irvine, CA, USA) is usually prescribed as 0.2% administered twice daily, totaling 0.4% per day.

Along with several previous studies demonstrating that chronic use of preserved eye drops causes significant damage to the ocular surface [13,17,21,24–26,56–58], we found that intra-group changes of the corneal and conjunctival staining scores at 12-week visits from the baseline score for each group showed different tendencies. The preserved group showed an increased corneal score in the ITT set and increased conjunctival score in both ITT and PP sets, which means an increased ocular surface defect of cornea and conjunctiva in the preserved brimonidine/timolol group. Also, we found that the TBUT was improved in the preservative-free group compared to preserved group, and the preserved group showed an increased OSDI score compared with the baseline at 12 weeks, while the preservative-free group showed consistently a decreased OSDI score which means better ocular surface status. These results imply that preservative-free brimonidine/timolol may reduce adverse effects of BAK on ocular surface. The higher patient adherence rate in the preservative-free group may be attributed to reduced BAK-related adverse effects, supported by the prior findings showing self-reported nonadherence rates of 32.0% for the preserved eye drops and 12.5% for the preservative-free eye drops [3].

Although inter-group change of the corneal and conjunctival staining and OSDI scores did not differ significantly between the preservative-free and preserved groups at 12-week visits, it does not mean the minimized adverse effect of BAK. A previous study comparing BAK-preserved latanoprost to BAK-free travoprost found that in the overall cohort of patients, mean OSDI scores at the 12-week time point were not statistically different, but significant improvement was seen in the subsets of patients with mild OSDI scores at baseline and patients who had long-term (more than 24 months) exposure to BAK-preserved latanoprost before entry into the study [24]. The latter finding suggests a cumulative effect of BAK, consistent with its persistence in ocular tissues [13]. On the contrary, the acute detrimental effect of BAK does not last long if the exposure time is a fairly short term. A recent study described that preserved latanoprost caused an acute decrease in the corneal epithelium at 1 min after the first instillation [56]. However, the decrease disappeared at 24 h after a once-daily application of the preserved latanoprost, which was also verified by scanning electron microscopy analyses [56]. This regenerative power in response to daily exposures to BAK may explain the lack of significant differences between the groups in ocular surface findings and OSDI scores during 4- and 12-week follow-up periods in this study. Alternatively, chronic changes from cumulative BAK toxicity might have been pronounced, potentially revealing a more significant detrimental effect on the corneal surface, if the follow-up period were longer [59]. On the other hands, intra-group changes of the corneal and conjunctival staining scores showed differences between the groups. In the preserved group, the corneal staining score continuously increased at 4 and 12 weeks compared to the baseline score, but in the preservative-free group, the scores were similar or showed decreasing tendency compared to the baseline score. This could possibly be related to the timing of the loss of corneal regenerative power due to the accumulation of BAK in the twice-daily use. Additionally, concerning the conjunctival staining score, there was a different trend between the groups. The preservative-free group showed no change at 4 and 12 weeks, while the preserved group showed an increased score at 12 weeks.

Ensuring patient adherence is a major concern for glaucoma treatment, as it significantly impacts patients' life-long medication use and influences the overall disease progression. In our study, adherence rates were consistently higher in the preservative-free group compared to the preserved group throughout the study period. Key differences between the two groups were differences in stinging/burning sensation and pain/soreness scores of drug tolerance, and easiness for instillation and storage of patient satisfaction scores. Participants using preservative-free brimonidine/timolol reported a lower stinging/burning sensation or pain/soreness score which could be related to ingredients in eye drop itself as mentioned above. Higher levels of patient satisfaction suggest that the single-dose container was both easy to use and convenient for storage. Although there is ongoing debate about whether elderly patients may struggle with opening rigid plastic containers of singe-dose units [60,61], this issue was not considered a significant hurdle for the newly developed preservative-free formulation. Moreover, patients can easily count the number of used or unused doses with the single-dose container system or keep the drug in desired locations, leading to better drug accessibility, resulting in convenient drug storage, another advantage of the preservative-free formulation in this study. Similar results were also reported in the previous study [26].

Since glaucoma is a chronic progressive disease property, long-term use of a glaucoma agent is often required. Initial treatment typically involves a single topical agent (monotherapy), but additional agents (combination therapy) are frequently needed to reach the target IOP [62–64]. Meanwhile, modern adjunctive therapy combines a β-receptor antagonists with another class of drug [65], and one of them is fixed-combination brimonidine/timolol which consists of brimonidine 0.2% and timolol 0.5%. In the Ocular Hypertension Treatment Study, 40% of treated subjects required more than one medication to achieve the therapeutic goal of 20% IOP reduction from baseline [62,64]. More than 75% of subjects in the medical treatment arm of the Collaborative Initial Glaucoma Treatment Study required at least two medications after 2 years [63]. Unfortunately, anti-glaucomatous eye drops often have significant adverse effects including OSD, which when combined with the silent nature of glaucoma leads to a high risk of low adherence if patients do not understand their disease and the importance of treatment [66]. Erb et al. [67] reported that the prevalence of dry eye disease in glaucoma was 52.6% and increased with age, the duration of glaucoma, and the number of eye drops used (1 eye drop 50.9%, 5 eye drops 66.7%). Therefore, use of fixed-combined drugs as treatment strategy to reduce the number of ophthalmic solutions may be reasonable while maintaining the comparable IOP-lowering effect and enhancing patient adherence.

This study has several limitations that should be considered when interpreting the findings. First, the relatively short follow-up period of 12 weeks may not fully capture the long-term effects of preservative-free versus preserved brimonidine/timolol on ocular surface health. Extended observation periods could provide a more comprehensive understanding of the chronic impacts on the ocular surface and adherence. Second, the dropout rate, although accounted for in the power calculation, led to a slightly uneven sample size between the groups, which may affect the statistical power in subgroup analyses. Additionally, the study was conducted across three institutions in South Korea, which may limit the generalizability of the results to populations with different demographic or environmental characteristics. Lastly, objective measures of inflammation, such as

MMP-9 levels, were not included. Future studies incorporating biomarkers for ocular surface inflammation may yield further insights into the differential effects of preserved and preservative-free formulations.

In sum, subjects with preservative-free brimonidine/timolol fixed-combination eyedrops showed better ocular surface status and higher patient adherence compared to the preserved formulation, especially in corneal/conjunctival staining scores and OSDI scores. Through serial investigations comparing patients' ocular surface status and adherence rate between the preserved and preservative-free eye drops [25,26], this study clearly demonstrates superiority of preservative-free eye drops on glaucoma patients in clinical application. Additionally, we discussed the influence of active pharmaceutical ingredients on ocular surface health, emphasizing the importance of considering both preservatives and active ingredients. Overall, our findings suggest that starting with preservative-free brimonidine/timolol rather than preserved formulation could be beneficial to improve the glaucoma drug adherence. Further studies with patients having different corneal properties and longer follow-up may be required to investigate the long-term effect of preservative-free and preserved medications in diverse settings.

Author Contributions: Conceptualization, S.R.; methodology, M.K. and S.R.; validation, M.K. and S.R.; writing—original draft preparation, M.K.; writing—review and editing, M.K., C.-K.L., J.S., D.K. and S.R.; visualization, M.K.; supervision, S.R.; project administration, S.R. All authors have read and agreed to the published version of the manuscript.

Funding: This research was funded by Hanlim Pharm, Seoul, Republic of Korea (Clinical Trial Protocol Number: BCT).

Institutional Review Board Statement: The study was approved by the institutional review boards (IRB) of CHA Bundang Medical Center (IRB number 2021-06-085), adhered to the tenets of the Declaration of Helsinki, and was registered on clinicaltrials.gov on 8 October 2021 (NCT06078592).

Informed Consent Statement: Informed consent was obtained from all subjects involved in the study.

Data Availability Statement: The data presented in this study are available on request from the corresponding author. The data are not publicly available due to privacy.

Conflicts of Interest: The authors declare no conflicts of interest.

References

1. Vermeire, E.; Hearnshaw, H.; Van Royen, P.; Denekens, J. Patient adherence to treatment: Three decades of research. A comprehensive review. *J. Clin. Pharm. Ther.* **2001**, *26*, 331–342. [CrossRef] [PubMed]
2. DiMatteo, M.R.; Giordani, P.J.; Lepper, H.S.; Croghan, T.W. Patient adherence and medical treatment outcomes: A meta-analysis. *Med. Care* **2002**, *40*, 794–811. [CrossRef]
3. Wolfram, C.; Stahlberg, E.; Pfeiffer, N. Patient-Reported Nonadherence with Glaucoma Therapy. *J. Ocul. Pharmacol. Ther.* **2019**, *35*, 223–228. [CrossRef] [PubMed]
4. Tapply, I.; Broadway, D.C. Improving adherence to topical medication in patients with glaucoma. *Patient Prefer. Adherence* **2021**, *15*, 1477–1489. [CrossRef]
5. Ha, A.; Jang, M.; Shim, S.R.; Kim, C.Y.; Chang, I.B.; Kim, Y.K. Interventions for glaucoma medication adherence improvement: A network meta-analysis of randomized controlled trials. *Ophthalmology* **2022**, *129*, 1294–1304. [CrossRef]
6. Tse, A.; Shah, M.; Jamal, N.; Shaikh, A. Glaucoma treatment adherence at a United Kingdom general practice. *Eye* **2016**, *30*, 1118–1122. [CrossRef]
7. Friedman, D.S.; Okeke, C.O.; Jampel, H.D.; Ying, G.-S.; Plyler, R.J.; Jiang, Y.; Quigley, H.A. Risk factors for poor adherence to eyedrops in electronically monitored patients with glaucoma. *Ophthalmology* **2009**, *116*, 1097–1105. [CrossRef]
8. Ung, C.; Zhang, E.; Alfaro, T.; Murakami, Y.; Zhang, M.; Seider, M.I.; Lin, S.C.; Singh, K. Glaucoma severity and medication adherence in a county hospital population. *Ophthalmology* **2013**, *120*, 1150–1157. [CrossRef]

9. Farkouh, A.; Frigo, P.; Czejka, M. Systemic side effects of eye drops: A pharmacokinetic perspective. *Clin. Ophthalmol.* **2016**, *10*, 2433–2441. [CrossRef]
10. Vaajanen, A.; Vapaatalo, H. A single drop in the eye–effects on the whole body? *Open Ophthalmol. J.* **2017**, *11*, 305. [CrossRef]
11. Müller, M. Syncope following ophthalmic administration in elderly patients: 3 case reports. *Reactions* **2006**, *1099*, 29.
12. Zanden, J.A.V.; Valuck, R.J.; Bunch, C.L.; Perlman, J.I.; Anderson, C.; Wortman, G.I. Systemic adverse effects of ophthalmic β-blockers. *Ann. Pharmacother.* **2001**, *35*, 1633–1637. [CrossRef]
13. Baudouin, C.; Labbe, A.; Liang, H.; Pauly, A.; Brignole-Baudouin, F. Preservatives in eyedrops: The good, the bad and the ugly. *Prog. Retin. Eye Res.* **2010**, *29*, 312–334. [CrossRef]
14. Charnock, C. Are multidose over-the-counter artificial tears adequately preserved? *Cornea* **2006**, *25*, 432–437. [CrossRef]
15. Baudouin, C.; Renard, J.P.; Nordmann, J.P.; Denis, P.; Lachkar, Y.; Sellem, E.; Rouland, J.F.; Jeanbat, V.; Bouee, S. Prevalence and risk factors for ocular surface disease among patients treated over the long term for glaucoma or ocular hypertension. *Eur. J. Ophthalmol.* **2013**, *23*, 47–54. [CrossRef]
16. Garcia-Feijoo, J.; Sampaolesi, J.R. A multicenter evaluation of ocular surface disease prevalence in patients with glaucoma. *Clin. Ophthalmol.* **2012**, *6*, 441–446. [CrossRef]
17. Leung, E.W.; Medeiros, F.A.; Weinreb, R.N. Prevalence of ocular surface disease in glaucoma patients. *J. Glaucoma* **2008**, *17*, 350–355. [CrossRef]
18. Pisella, P.J.; Pouliquen, P.; Baudouin, C. Prevalence of ocular symptoms and signs with preserved and preservative free glaucoma medication. *Br. J. Ophthalmol.* **2002**, *86*, 418–423. [CrossRef]
19. Goldstein, M.H.; Silva, F.Q.; Blender, N.; Tran, T.; Vantipalli, S. Ocular benzalkonium chloride exposure: Problems and solutions. *Eye* **2022**, *36*, 361–368. [CrossRef]
20. Wu, J.-H.; Wang, T.-H.; Huang, J.-Y.; Su, C.-C. Ocular surface disease in glaucoma patients randomized to benzalkonium chloride-containing latanoprost and preservative-free bimatoprost. *J. Ocul. Pharmacol. Ther.* **2021**, *37*, 556–564. [CrossRef]
21. Uusitalo, H.; Chen, E.; Pfeiffer, N.; Brignole-Baudouin, F.; Kaarniranta, K.; Leino, M.; Puska, P.; Palmgren, E.; Hamacher, T.; Hofmann, G.; et al. Switching from a preserved to a preservative-free prostaglandin preparation in topical glaucoma medication. *Acta Ophthalmol.* **2010**, *88*, 329–336. [CrossRef]
22. Rossi, G.C.M.; Blini, M.; Scudeller, L.; Ricciardelli, G.; Depolo, L.; Amisano, A.; Bossolesi, L.; Pasinetti, G.M.; Bianchi, P.E. Effect of preservative-free tafluprost on keratocytes, sub-basal nerves, and endothelium: A single-blind one-year confocal study on naïve or treated glaucoma and hypertensive patients versus a control group. *J. Ocul. Pharmacol. Ther.* **2013**, *29*, 821–825. [CrossRef]
23. Kaštelan, S.; Tomić, M.; Salopek-Rabatić, J. How ocular surface disease impacts the glaucoma treatment outcome. *BioMed Res. Int.* **2013**, *2013*, 696328. [CrossRef]
24. Katz, G.; Springs, C.L.; Craven, E.R.; Montecchi-Palmer, M. Ocular surface disease in patients with glaucoma or ocular hypertension treated with either BAK-preserved latanoprost or BAK-free travoprost. *Clin. Ophthalmol.* **2010**, *4*, 1253–1261. [CrossRef]
25. Kim, D.W.; Shin, J.; Lee, C.K.; Kim, M.; Lee, S.; Rho, S. Comparison of ocular surface assessment and adherence between preserved and preservative-free latanoprost in glaucoma: A parallel-grouped randomized trial. *Sci. Rep.* **2021**, *11*, 14971. [CrossRef]
26. Kim, K.E.; Lee, C.K.; Shin, J.; Kim, Y.; Rho, S. Comparisons of efficacy and safety between preserved and preservative-free brimonidine tartrate in glaucoma and ocular hypertension: A parallel-grouped, randomized trial. *Sci. Rep.* **2023**, *13*, 5700. [CrossRef]
27. Gardiner, S.K.; Fortune, B.; Demirel, S. Localized changes in retinal nerve fiber layer thickness as a predictor of localized functional change in glaucoma. *Am. J. Ophthalmol.* **2016**, *170*, 75–82. [CrossRef]
28. Badalà, F.; Nouri-Mahdavi, K.; Raoof, D.A.; Leeprechanon, N.; Law, S.K.; Caprioli, J. Optic disk and nerve fiber layer imaging to detect glaucoma. *Am. J. Ophthalmol.* **2007**, *144*, 724–732. [CrossRef]
29. Holladay, J.T. Proper method for calculating average visual acuity. *J. Refract. Surg.* **1997**, *13*, 388–391. [CrossRef]
30. Ehlers, N.; Bramsen, T.; Sperling, S. Applanation tonometry and central corneal thickness. *Acta Ophthalmol.* **1975**, *53*, 34–43. [CrossRef]
31. Moses, R.A. The Goldmann applanation tonometer. *Am. J. Ophthalmol.* **1958**, *46*, 865–869. [CrossRef] [PubMed]
32. Doughty, M.J.; Zaman, M.L. Human corneal thickness and its impact on intraocular pressure measures: A review and meta-analysis approach. *Surv. Ophthalmol.* **2000**, *44*, 367–408. [CrossRef]
33. Faschinger, C.; Hommer, A. *Gonioscopy*; Springer Science & Business Media: Berlin/Heidelberg, Germany, 2012.
34. Sugar, H.S. Gonioscopy and glaucoma. *Arch. Ophthalmol.* **1941**, *25*, 674–717. [CrossRef]
35. Heijl, A.; Lindgren, G.; Olsson, J. Normal variability of static perimetric threshold values across the central visual field. *Arch. Ophthalmol.* **1987**, *105*, 1544–1549. [CrossRef]

36. Hasanreisoglu, M.; Priel, E.; Naveh, L.; Lusky, M.; Weinberger, D.; Benjamini, Y.; Gaton, D.D. Digital versus film stereophotography for assessment of the optic nerve head in glaucoma and glaucoma suspect patients. *J. Glaucoma* **2013**, *22*, 238–242. [CrossRef]
37. Rao, H.L.; Pradhan, Z.S.; Suh, M.H.; Moghimi, S.; Mansouri, K.; Weinreb, R.N. Optical coherence tomography angiography in glaucoma. *J. Glaucoma* **2020**, *29*, 312–321. [CrossRef]
38. Van Melkebeke, L.; Barbosa-Breda, J.; Huygens, M.; Stalmans, I. Optical coherence tomography angiography in glaucoma: A review. *Ophthalmic Res.* **2018**, *60*, 139–151. [CrossRef]
39. Spaide, R.F.; Klancnik, J.M.; Cooney, M.J. Retinal vascular layers imaged by fluorescein angiography and optical coherence tomography angiography. *JAMA Ophthalmol.* **2015**, *133*, 45–50. [CrossRef]
40. Bron, A.J.; Evans, V.E.; Smith, J.A. Grading of corneal and conjunctival staining in the context of other dry eye tests. *Cornea* **2003**, *22*, 640–650. [CrossRef]
41. Begley, C.; Caffery, B.; Chalmers, R.; Situ, P.; Simpson, T.; Nelson, J.D. Review and analysis of grading scales for ocular surface staining. *Ocul. Surf.* **2019**, *17*, 208–220. [CrossRef]
42. Schiffman, R.M.; Christianson, M.D.; Jacobsen, G.; Hirsch, J.D.; Reis, B.L. Reliability and validity of the ocular surface disease index. *Arch. Ophthalmol.* **2000**, *118*, 615–621. [CrossRef] [PubMed]
43. Efron, N. Grading scales for contact lens complications. *Ophthalmic Physiol. Opt.* **1998**, *18*, 182–186. [CrossRef] [PubMed]
44. Misiuk-Hojlo, M.; Pomorska, M.; Mulak, M.; Rekas, M.; Wierzbowska, J.; Prost, M.; Wasyluk, J.; Lubinski, W.; Podboraczynska-Jodko, K.; Romaniuk, W.; et al. The RELIEF study: Tolerability and efficacy of preservative-free latanoprost in the treatment of glaucoma or ocular hypertension. *Eur. J. Ophthalmol.* **2019**, *29*, 210–215. [CrossRef] [PubMed]
45. Delval, L.; Baudouin, C.; Gabisson, P.; Alliot, E.; Vincent, B.; Group, D.S. Safety and efficacy of unpreserved timolol 0.1% gel in patients controlled by preserved latanoprost with signs of ocular intolerance. *J. Français D'ophtalmologie* **2013**, *36*, 316–323. [CrossRef]
46. Guenoun, J.M.; Baudouin, C.; Rat, P.; Pauly, A.; Warnet, J.M.; Brignole-Baudouin, F. In Vitro study of inflammatory potential and toxicity profile of latanoprost, travoprost, and bimatoprost in conjunctiva-derived epithelial cells. *Investig. Ophthalmol. Vis. Sci.* **2005**, *46*, 2444–2450. [CrossRef]
47. Guenoun, J.M.; Baudouin, C.; Rat, P.; Pauly, A.; Warnet, J.M.; Brignole-Baudouin, F. In Vitro comparison of cytoprotective and antioxidative effects of latanoprost, travoprost, and bimatoprost on conjunctiva-derived epithelial cells. *Investig. Ophthalmol. Vis. Sci.* **2005**, *46*, 4594–4599. [CrossRef]
48. Pisella, P.J.; Debbasch, C.; Hamard, P.; Creuzot-Garcher, C.; Rat, P.; Brignole, F.; Baudouin, C. Conjunctival proinflammatory and proapoptotic effects of latanoprost and preserved and unpreserved timolol: An Ex Vivo and In Vitro study. *Investig. Ophthalmol. Vis. Sci.* **2004**, *45*, 1360–1368. [CrossRef]
49. Yu, A.L.; Fuchshofer, R.; Kampik, A.; Welge-Lussen, U. Effects of oxidative stress in trabecular meshwork cells are reduced by prostaglandin analogues. *Investig. Ophthalmol. Vis. Sci.* **2008**, *49*, 4872–4880. [CrossRef]
50. Sherwood, M.B.; Craven, E.R.; Chou, C.; DuBiner, H.B.; Batoosingh, A.L.; Schiffman, R.M.; Whitcup, S.M. Twice-daily 0.2% brimonidine-0.5% timolol fixed-combination therapy vs monotherapy with timolol or brimonidine in patients with glaucoma or ocular hypertension: A 12-month randomized trial. *Arch. Ophthalmol.* **2006**, *124*, 1230–1238. [CrossRef]
51. Adkins, J.C.; Balfour, J.A. Brimonidine. A review of its pharmacological properties and clinical potential in the management of open-angle glaucoma and ocular hypertension. *Drugs Aging* **1998**, *12*, 225–241. [CrossRef]
52. Leier, C.V.; Baker, N.D.; Weber, P.A. Cardiovascular effects of ophthalmic timolol. *Ann. Intern. Med.* **1986**, *104*, 197–199. [CrossRef]
53. Nino, J.; Tahvanainen, K.; Uusitalo, H.; Turjanmaa, V.; Hutri-Kahonen, N.; Kaila, T.; Ropo, A.; Kuusela, T.; Kahonen, M. Cardiovascular effects of ophthalmic 0.5% timolol aqueous solution and 0.1% timolol hydrogel. *Clin. Physiol. Funct. Imaging* **2002**, *22*, 271–278. [CrossRef]
54. Stewart, W.C.; Stewart, J.A.; Jackson, A.L. Cardiovascular effects of timolol maleate, brimonidine or brimonidine/timolol maleate in concomitant therapy. *Acta Ophthalmol. Scand.* **2002**, *80*, 277–281. [CrossRef]
55. Na, K.H.; Yoo, C.; Park, J.H.; Kim, Y.Y. Eye Drop Dispenser Type and Medication Possession Ratio in Patients with Glaucoma: Single-Use Containers Versus Multiple-Use Bottles. *Am. J. Ophthalmol.* **2018**, *188*, 9–18. [CrossRef]
56. Inoue, D.; Mohamed, Y.H.; Uematsu, M.; Kitaoka, T. Corneal damage and its recovery after instillation of preservative-free versus preserved latanoprost eye drops. *Cutan. Ocul. Toxicol.* **2020**, *39*, 158–164. [CrossRef]
57. Chen, X.; Sullivan, D.A.; Sullivan, A.G.; Kam, W.R.; Liu, Y. Toxicity of cosmetic preservatives on human ocular surface and adnexal cells. *Exp. Eye Res.* **2018**, *170*, 188–197. [CrossRef]
58. De Saint Jean, M.; Debbasch, C.; Brignole, F.; Rat, P.; Warnet, J.M.; Baudouin, C. Toxicity of preserved and unpreserved antiglaucoma topical drugs in an In Vitro model of conjunctival cells. *Curr. Eye Res.* **2000**, *20*, 85–94. [CrossRef]

59. Hedengran, A.; Steensberg, A.T.; Virgili, G.; Azuara-Blanco, A.; Kolko, M. Efficacy and safety evaluation of benzalkonium chloride preserved eye-drops compared with alternatively preserved and preservative-free eye-drops in the treatment of glaucoma: A systematic review and meta-analysis. *Br. J. Ophthalmol.* **2020**, *104*, 1512–1518. [CrossRef]
60. Dietlein, T.S.; Jordan, J.F.; Luke, C.; Schild, A.; Dinslage, S.; Krieglstein, G.K. Self-application of single-use eyedrop containers in an elderly population: Comparisons with standard eyedrop bottle and with younger patients. *Acta Ophthalmol.* **2008**, *86*, 856–859. [CrossRef]
61. Parkkari, M.; Latvala, T.; Ropo, A. Handling test of eye drop dispenser--comparison of unit-dose pipettes with conventional eye drop bottles. *J. Ocul. Pharmacol. Ther.* **2010**, *26*, 273–276. [CrossRef]
62. Kass, M.A.; Heuer, D.K.; Higginbotham, E.J.; Parrish, R.K.; Khanna, C.L.; Brandt, J.D.; Soltau, J.B.; Johnson, C.A.; Keltner, J.L.; Huecker, J.B.; et al. Assessment of Cumulative Incidence and Severity of Primary Open-Angle Glaucoma Among Participants in the Ocular Hypertension Treatment Study After 20 Years of Follow-up. *JAMA Ophthalmol.* **2021**, *139*, 558–566. [CrossRef] [PubMed]
63. Janz, N.K.; Wren, P.A.; Lichter, P.R.; Musch, D.C.; Gillespie, B.W.; Guire, K.E.; Mills, R.P.; Group, C.S. The Collaborative Initial Glaucoma Treatment Study: Interim quality of life findings after initial medical or surgical treatment of glaucoma. *Ophthalmology* **2001**, *108*, 1954–1965. [CrossRef] [PubMed]
64. Kass, M.A.; Heuer, D.K.; Higginbotham, E.J.; Johnson, C.A.; Keltner, J.L.; Miller, J.P.; Parrish, R.K., 2nd; Wilson, M.R.; Gordon, M.O. The Ocular Hypertension Treatment Study: A randomized trial determines that topical ocular hypotensive medication delays or prevents the onset of primary open-angle glaucoma. *Arch. Ophthalmol.* **2002**, *120*, 701–713; discussion 730–829. [CrossRef] [PubMed]
65. Fechtner, R.D.; Realini, T. Fixed combinations of topical glaucoma medications. *Curr. Opin. Ophthalmol.* **2004**, *15*, 132–135. [CrossRef]
66. Kalouda, P.; Keskini, C.; Anastasopoulos, E.; Topouzis, F. Achievements and Limits of Current Medical Therapy of Glaucoma. *Dev. Ophthalmol.* **2017**, *59*, 1–14. [CrossRef]
67. Erb, C.; Gast, U.; Schremmer, D. German register for glaucoma patients with dry eye. I. Basic outcome with respect to dry eye. *Graefes Arch. Clin. Exp. Ophthalmol.* **2008**, *246*, 1593–1601. [CrossRef]

Journal of
Clinical Medicine

MDPI

Article

Potential Causal Association Between Atrial Fibrillation/Flutter and Primary Open-Angle Glaucoma: A Two-Sample Mendelian Randomisation Study

Young Lee † and Je Hyun Seo *,†

Veterans Medical Research Institute, Veterans Health Service Medical Center, Seoul 05368, Republic of Korea; lyou7688@gmail.com

* Correspondence: jazmin2@naver.com; Tel.: +82-2-2225-1445

† These authors contributed equally to this work.

Abstract: Background: A few studies have reported controversial relationships between atrial fibrillation/flutter (AF/L) and primary open-angle glaucoma (POAG). This study aimed to investigate the potential causal relationship between AF/L and POAG. **Methods**: Single-nucleotide polymorphisms associated with exposure to AF/L were selected as instrumental variables with significance ($p < 5.0 \times 10^{-8}$) from a genome-wide association study (GWAS) by FinnGen. The GWAS summary of POAG from the UK Biobank was used as the outcome dataset. A two-sample Mendelian randomisation (MR) study was performed to assess the causal effects of AF/L on POAG. In addition, potential confounders, including hypertension, autoimmune hyperthyroidism, sleep apnoea, and alcohol use disorder, were assessed using multivariable MR analysis. **Results:** There was a significant causal association of AF/L with POAG (odds ratio [OR] = 1.26, 95% confidence interval [CI] = 1.07–1.48, $p = 0.005$ using inverse-variance weighting [IVW]). Multivariable MR analysis confirmed a causal association of AF/L with POAG (OR = 1.24, 95% CI = 1.02–1.51, $p = 0.034$ using IVW), but hypertension, hyperthyroidism, sleep apnoea and alcohol use disorder did not show significant causal associations with POAG (all $p > 0.05$). **Conclusions:** This established causal relationship between AF/L and POAG supports the need for further investigation into the role of AF/L as a possible risk factor for POAG. Further research is required to confirm these findings.

Keywords: primary open-angle glaucoma; mendelian randomisation; atrial fibrillation; atrial flutter; sleep apnoea; single-nucleotide polymorphisms

1. Introduction

Primary open-angle glaucoma (POAG), a major cause of permanent vision loss, is a progressive optic neuropathy characterised by the degeneration of retinal ganglion cells and their axons [1]. Its pathogenesis remains unclear, despite the established roles of multiple factors in its pathophysiology. Elevated intraocular pressure (IOP) is a major risk factor for POAG [2], although the precise mechanisms underlying glaucomatous optic neuropathy and the associated visual field loss remain unclear [1]. However, reports indicate that lowering IOP with long-acting drug delivery reduces the risk of glaucoma progression, highlighting that IOP is a critical factor in glaucoma [3]. Studies identifying the causal risk factors for POAG may enable the early detection and prevention of glaucoma; consequently, they form the foundation for research in ophthalmology. Several risk factors, such as ageing, hypoxia, neuroprotection, and environmental factors, have been suggested as contributing to the pathogenesis of POAG [1,4–9]. Minor injuries from repeated reperfusion, such as fluctuating IOP or disrupted autoregulation, may eventually cause oxidative stress and glaucomatous damage [10]. Cardiovascular disorders, including vasospasm, hypertension, and hypotension, are also potential risk factors for glaucoma [11].

Atrial fibrillation (AF) and atrial flutter (AFL) are disorders of significant importance to public health, especially when considering their associations with ischaemic stroke and heart failure [12,13]. AF is the most prevalent type of cardiac arrhythmia, caused by aberrant electrical activity within the atria of the heart, leading to fibrillation. AFL is similar to AF, but the rapid upper-chamber cardiac arrhythmias encountered in clinical practice are often more regular [14]. Additionally, many patients with AFL develop AF over time [15]. Recent advances in the understanding of the unique electrophysiological processes underlying AF and AFL have led to anatomy-based treatment approaches. Owing to their mechanistic similarities, AF and AFL (AF/L) are often classified and studied together. AF prevalence ranges from 2% in the general population to 10–12% in those aged ≥80 years. AF/L presents as an erratic heartbeat that may cause instability in ocular perfusion pressure. AF/L plays a significant role in heart failure, stroke, cardiovascular morbidity, and sudden death. However, the associations between AF/L, as a major cardiovascular disease, and ophthalmological diseases have not been intensively examined. A recent analysis from the Ural Eye and Medical Study showed that AF/L was not associated with major ocular diseases, including glaucoma ($p = 0.90$) [16]. However, Flammer et al. suggested that ischaemia and reperfusion damage caused by unstable ocular perfusion may play a role in the vascular pathophysiology of POAG [17]. An observational study also revealed that patients with normal-tension glaucoma had a higher AF incidence than controls ($p = 0.022$) [18]. Another recent longitudinal study evaluating the association of AF and glaucoma using Korean National Health Insurance data determined that AF increased the risk of developing glaucoma (hazard ratio = 1.31; 95% confidence interval [CI] = 1.15–1.48) [19]. Evidently, research on the relationship between AF and glaucoma is not enough.

Mendelian randomisation (MR) is a genetic epidemiological technique that uses genetic variants associated with potential risk factors (exposures) as instrumental variables (IVs) to assess their causal effects on disease outcomes [20,21]. Several studies have used MR to investigate glaucoma and its potential risk factors [22–24]. However, no MR studies have assessed the association between AF/L and POAG. Therefore, this study aimed to analyse the association between AF/L and POAG using univariate MR analysis and to conduct multivariate MR analysis to account for potential confounding factors, such as hypertension, hyperthyroidism, sleep apnoea, and alcohol use disorder. To achieve this goal, a two-sample MR technique was used to examine the causal effects of AF/L on POAG, utilising summary statistics from FinnGen [25] for exposures and from the UK Biobank (UKB) for outcomes [26].

2. Materials and Methods

2.1. Study Design

The study protocol was approved by the Institutional Review Board of the Veterans Health Service Medical Center (approval number. 2023-12-030), and owing to the retrospective study design, the requirement for informed consent was waived. This study was conducted in accordance with the principles of the Declaration of Helsinki.

2.2. Data Sources

The analytical study design used to investigate the causal relationship between AF/L and POAG is presented in Figure 1. The following summary datasets were used: exposure data from the FinnGen genome-wide association study (GWAS) for AF/L, which included 237,690 participants (45,766 cases vs. 191,924 controls), and outcome data from the UKB POAG GWAS, which included 456,351 participants (654 cases vs. 455,697 controls). To assess the causal relationship between AF/L and glaucoma, additional FinnGen data from the following participant types were incorporated in the multivariable MR analysis to assess potential confounders: 377,209 participants with hypertension (111,581 cases vs. 265,626 controls), 281,683 participants with autoimmune hyperthyroidism (1828 cases vs. 279,855 controls), 375,657 participants with sleep apnoea (38,998 cases vs. 336,659 controls) and 377,277 participants with alcohol use disorder (15,715 cases vs. 361,562 controls). Detailed sources of the summary data are presented in Table 1.

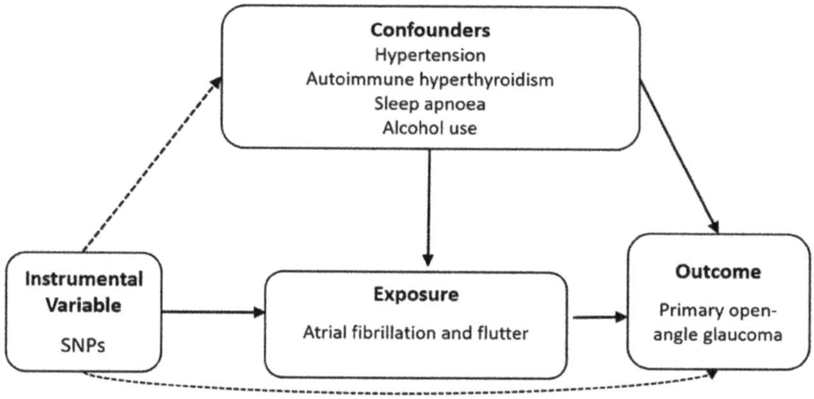

Figure 1. Diagram of two-sample Mendelian randomisation analysis. Solid lines indicate an association, while dashed lines indicate none. Abbreviation: SNP, single-nucleotide polymorphism.

Table 1. Summary statistics of data sources.

Traits	Data Source	No. of Participants	Population	No. of Variants	Reference
Atrial fibrillation and flutter	FinnGen	237,690 (45,766 cases + 191,924 controls)	European (Finland)	20,164,886	[27]
Hypertension	FinnGen	377,209 (111,581 cases + 265,626 controls)	European (Finland)	20,170,234	
Autoimmune hyperthyroidism	FinnGen	281,683 (1828 cases + 279,855 controls)	European (Finland)	20,167,370	
Sleep apnoea	FinnGen	375,657 (38,998 cases + 336,659 controls)	European (Finland)	20,170,208	
Alcohol use disorder, ICD-based	FinnGen	377,277 (15,715 cases + 361,562 controls)	European (Finland)	20,170,236	
Primary open-angle glaucoma	UKB	456,351 (654 cases + 455,697 controls)	European (UK)	11,831,932	[28]

Abbreviations: ICD, International Classification of Diseases; UK, United Kingdom; UKB, UK Biobank.

2.3. Selection of the Genetic IVs

The study used single-nucleotide polymorphisms (SNPs) associated with exposure at the GWAS significance threshold ($p < 5.0 \times 10^{-8}$) as IVs. To maintain the independence of each IV, SNPs were selected after pruning for linkage disequilibrium ($R^2 < 0.001$, clumping distance = 10,000 kb). Data from the 1000 Genomes Phase III European database were used as a reference to calculate linkage disequilibrium during the clumping process. The F-statistic was calculated using the formula

$$F = R^2(n-2)/(1-R^2)$$

where n represents the sample size, and R^2 is the proportion of variance in the exposure explained by the genetic variants [29]. An F-statistic >10 suggests no indication of weak instrument bias [30]. For the multivariable MR analysis, the strength of the IVs was evaluated using conditional F-statistics, with values of >10 indicating sufficient instrument strength for the analysis [31].

2.4. MR Analysis

In this study, a two-sample MR approach with SNPs was used as IVs to investigate the causal effect of AF/L on POAG. For valid causal inference, IVs were required to meet the following three assumptions: (1) SNPs should be strongly associated with AF/L; (2) SNPs should not be associated with confounders of the AF/L–POAG relationship; and (3) SNPs should influence POAG exclusively through AF/L, with no evidence of directional horizontal pleiotropy. Our primary analytical method was inverse-variance weighting (IVW) with a multiplicative random effects model [30,32,33]. The IVW approach is most efficient when all genetic variations satisfy the three IV assumptions [34]. Recognising the potential bias that may arise from invalid IVs if the assumptions were not fully met, sensitivity analyses were conducted using the weighted median method [35] and MR-Egger regression [36,37]. The weighted median method can provide a consistent estimate even if more than 50% of the IVs are invalid [35]. MR-Egger regression, which is less sensitive to pleiotropy, estimates the average horizontal pleiotropy through its intercept, providing an unbiased estimate of the causal effect [36]. Further, MR-Egger analysis with simulation extrapolation (SIMEX) was employed as it allows bias correction in scenarios where the 'no measurement error' assumption is violated, such as when the I^2 value is <90% [37]. To assess heterogeneity and potential pleiotropy, we used Cochran's Q statistics from the IVW method and Rücker's Q statistics from the MR-Egger analysis [32,38]. We also employed the MR pleiotropy residual sum and outlier (MR-PRESSO) [39] test and conducted a 'leave-one-SNP-out' analysis to identify the influence of potentially pleiotropic SNPs on our estimates. Considering that hypertension, autoimmune hyperthyroidism, sleep apnoea, and alcohol use disorder are common risk factors for POAG, multivariable MR IVW [20] and MR-Egger [40] approaches were used to adjust for these factors and isolate the effects of AF/L on POAG. The Q_A statistic, a modification of Cochran's Q, was used to assess the heterogeneity and potential pleiotropy among IVs [31]. When the conditional F-statistic or Q_A statistics indicated the presence of weak instruments or potential pleiotropy, the Q-minimisation approach (Q-het) was applied to estimate robust causal associations, supplementing the MVMR-IVW approach. The standard errors were calculated using the bootstrap method [31]. For exposures with overlapping samples, covariances for the effect of each SNP on each exposure were required to calculate the conditional F-statistic and Q_A statistics [31]. One approach to obtain these covariances is to use a phenotypic correlation matrix [31], which can be derived from the intercept of the bivariate LD score regression [41–43]. Causal effects are expressed as odds ratios (ORs) with 95% CIs. Statistical significance was established at a two-tailed p-value of <0.05. All MR analyses were performed using the TwoSampleMR, MVMR, Mendelian randomisation, and SIMEX packages in R version 3.6.3 (R Core Team, Vienna, Austria).

3. Results

3.1. Genetic IVs in Univariable MR

In the MR study, 85 SNPs that were significant at the GWAS level and were independent of each other were selected to serve as IVs. The F-statistic values for all the selected SNPs exceeded 10, with a mean value of 114.53, confirming that they were strong instruments. Detailed information on the IVs is provided in Supplementary Table S1. According to the results, the assumption of no measurement error was satisfied, with an I^2 value of 97.93% (Table 2). Heterogeneity among the IVs was evaluated using Cochran's Q test from the IVW method and Rücker's Q' test from the MR-Egger analysis and found no significant heterogeneity ($p = 0.338$ for Cochran's Q and $p = 0.312$ for Rücker's Q'; Table 2). Horizontal pleiotropy was assessed using the MR-PRESSO global test and MR-Egger regression, both with and without SIMEX adjustments; the MR-PRESSO global test indicated no significant pleiotropic effects ($p = 0.338$), and the MR-Egger intercepts showed no evidence of horizontal pleiotropy (intercept = 0.004, $p = 0.797$ without SIMEX; Intercept = 0.004, $p = 0.848$ with SIMEX), as shown in Table 2. Given that the F-statistic indicated no evidence of weak instrument bias, the I^2 statistic exceeded 90, and Cochran's Q test was not significant, the IVW method was selected for primary analysis because of its superior statistical power when core MR assumptions were satisfied [44].

Table 2. Heterogeneity and horizontal pleiotropy of instrumental variables.

Exposure				Heterogeneity			Horizontal Pleiotropy			
							MR-Egger		MR-Egger (SIMEX)	
	N	F	I^2 (%)	p-Value *	p-Value #	p-Value †	Intercept, β (SE)	p-Value	Intercept, β (SE)	p-Value
Atrial fibrillation and flutter	85	114.53	97.93	0.338	0.312	0.338	0.004 (0.017)	0.797	0.004 (0.018)	0.848

Abbreviations: β, beta coefficient; F, mean F-statistic; MR, Mendelian randomisation; N, number of instruments; PRESSO, pleiotropy residual sum and outlier; SE, standard error; SIMEX, simulation extrapolation. * Cochran's Q test from the inverse-variance weighting. # Rücker's Q' test from MR-Egger. † MR-PRESSO global test.

3.2. Univariable MR for the Causal Effects of AF/L on POAG

We explored the potential causal relationship between AF/L and POAG by employing 85 SNPs as IVs in a univariable MR analysis. The results, displayed in Figure 2, indicate that AF/L increases the risk of POAG according to the IVW method (OR =1.26, 95% CI = 1.07–1.48, p = 0.005). The weighted median approach revealed a similar trend, though it did not achieve statistical significance (OR = 1.25, 95% CI = 0.98–1.60, p = 0.068). No significant causal relationship was observed with the MR-Egger method, with or without SIMEX adjustment (OR = 1.20, 95% CI = 0.84–1.74, p = 0.323 without SIMEX; OR = 1.22, 95% CI = 0.82–1.81, p = 0.329 with SIMEX). Figure 3 displays a scatter plot of the effects of SNPs on AF/L and their corresponding effects on POAG. The leave-one-out analysis corroborated the primary IVW MR findings, as depicted in Figure 4.

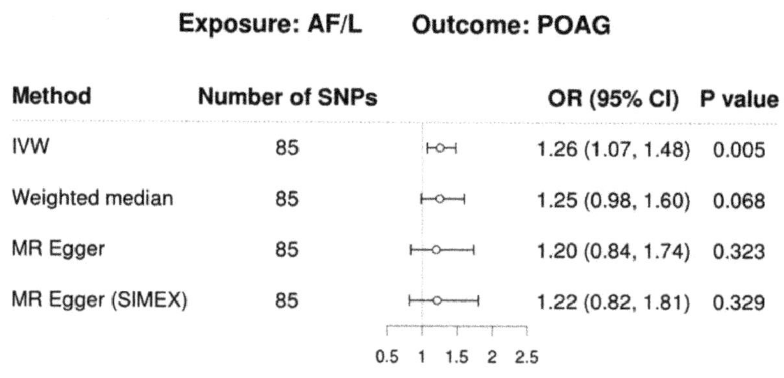

Figure 2. Forest plot of causal association of AF/L with POAG. The plot presents causal effect estimates from various MR methods, including IVW, MR-Egger, and MR-Egger with SIMEX correction. Each method is represented with its corresponding causal estimate and 95% CI. The x-axis indicates the OR for POAG associated with the presence of AF/L. Odds ratios greater than 1 suggest that AF/L increases the risk of POAG. Abbreviations: AF/L, atrial fibrillation and flutter; CI, confidence interval; OR, odds ratio; SNP, single-nucleotide polymorphism; IVW, inverse-variance weighting; MR, Mendelian randomisation; POAG, primary open-angle glaucoma; SIMEX, simulation extrapolation.

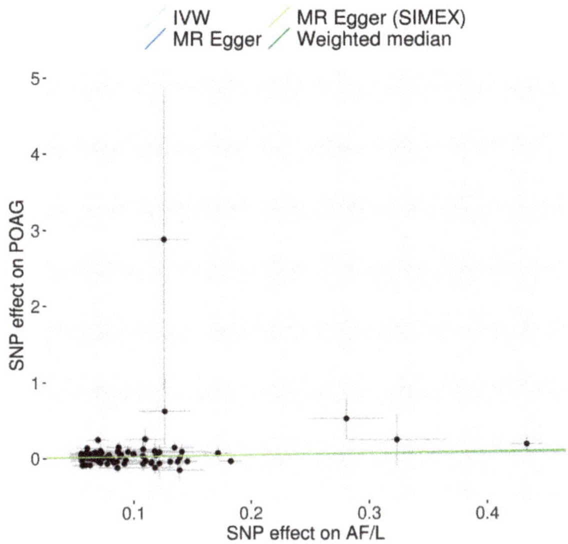

Figure 3. Scatterplot of MR tests showing the effect of AF/L on POAG. Each dot corresponds to an SNP, with the x-axis representing the association between the SNP and the exposure and the y-axis representing the association between the SNP and the outcome. The regression lines are colour-coded: light blue for IVW, dark blue for MR-Egger, light green for MR-Egger (SIMEX), and dark green for the Weighted Median method. The slope of each line indicates the causal effect estimate obtained through the respective method. Abbreviations: MR, Mendelian randomisation; AF/L, atrial fibrillation and flutter; IVW, inverse-variance weighting; SIMEX, simulation extrapolation; SNP, single-nucleotide polymorphism; POAG, primary open-angle glaucoma.

3.3. Multivariable MR for the Causal Effects of AF/L on POAG

In the multivariable MR analysis (controlled for hypertension, autoimmune hyperthyroidism, sleep apnoea, and alcohol use disorder), the association between AF/L and POAG remained significant (IVW OR = 1.24, 95% CI = 1.02–1.51, p = 0.034), as presented in Table 3 (Model 1). Hypertension, autoimmune hyperthyroidism, sleep apnoea, and alcohol use disorder were not significantly associated with POAG in Model 1. The causal effects estimated from the multivariate MR-Egger results were consistent with those of the IVW analysis (Table 3). The Q_A statistic for Model 1 was 211.99, with a p-value of 0.192, indicating no substantial heterogeneity among the IVs. The conditional F-statistics for autoimmune hyperthyroidism, sleep apnoea, and alcohol use disorder were below the conventional threshold of 10 (F = 4.08, 3.19, and 3.21, respectively), indicating potentially weak instruments for these exposures. In contrast, the conditional F-statistics for AF/L and hypertension were above 10 (F = 22.48 and 14.16, respectively), suggesting sufficient instrument strength for these variables. Given the potential bias introduced by weak instruments, we performed an additional multivariate MR analysis (Model 2) that included only AF/L and hypertension, which had conditional F-statistics above the threshold of 10. In Model 2, the association between AF/L and POAG remained significant (IVW OR = 1.24, 95% CI = 1.02–1.52, p = 0.032), consistent with the findings from Model 1. Hypertension continued to show no significant association with POAG in Model 2 (IVW OR = 0.90, 95% CI = 0.69–1.18, p = 0.449). The Q_A statistic for Model 2 was 212.86, with a p-value of 0.133, indicating no evidence of heterogeneity. To address potentially weak instruments, we also performed an IVW analysis with Q-minimisation (Q-het) for Model 1. The results of this analysis are presented in Supplementary Table S2 and are consistent with the standard IVW results for AF/L (OR = 1.38, 95% CI = 1.02–2.05).

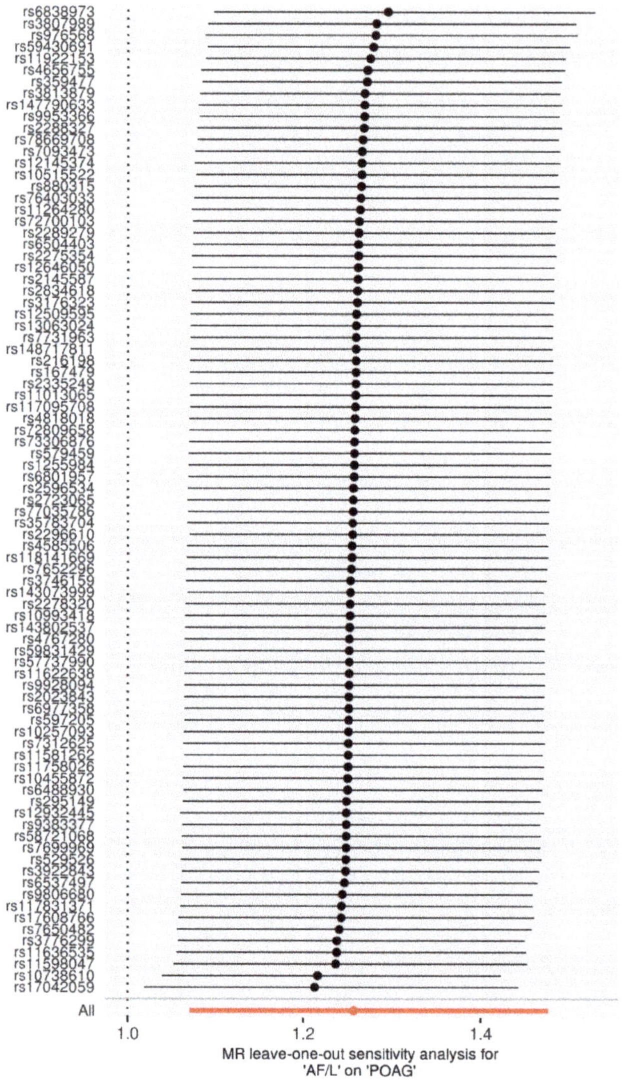

Figure 4. Leave-one-out plot in univariable MR analysis for the effect of AF/L on POAG. Each black dot represents the OR estimate of the causal effect after excluding a specific SNP, with the horizontal line around each dot indicating the corresponding 95% CI. The red dot and horizontal line represent the overall causal estimate (OR and CI) calculated using all SNPs. The *x*-axis represents ORs, where values greater than 1 suggest that AF/L increases the risk of POAG. Abbreviations: MR, Mendelian randomisation; AF/L, atrial fibrillation and flutter; POAG, primary open-angle glaucoma; OR, odds ratio; CI, confidence interval.

Table 3. Multivariable MR analysis.

Exposures	Conditional *F*	IVW		MR-Egger	
		OR (95% CI)	*p*-Value	OR (95% CI)	*p*-Value
Model 1					
Atrial fibrillation and flutter	22.48	1.24 (1.02, 1.51)	0.034	1.24 (1.02, 1.51)	0.034
Hypertension	14.16	1.00 (0.74, 1.34)	0.984	1.00 (0.74, 1.34)	0.983
Autoimmune hyperthyroidism	4.08	1.03 (0.91, 1.17)	0.617	1.04 (0.90, 1.20)	0.607
Sleep apnoea	3.19	0.60 (0.33, 1.09)	0.092	0.60 (0.33, 1.09)	0.094
Alcohol use disorder, ICD-based	3.21	1.09 (0.80, 1.48)	0.596	1.09 (0.80, 1.48)	0.595
Model 2					
Atrial fibrillation and flutter	20.75	1.24 (1.02, 1.52)	0.032	1.28 (1.04, 1.57)	0.019
Hypertension	25.84	0.90 (0.69, 1.18)	0.449	1.12 (0.69, 1.83)	0.637

Abbreviations: MR, Mendelian randomisation; *F*, *F*-statistic; IVW, inverse-variance weighting; OR, odds ratio; CI, confidence interval; ICD, International Classification of Diseases.

4. Discussion

The findings suggest a potential causal relationship between AF/L and POAG. Moreover, after controlling for the risk factors for AF/L and POAG, including hypertension, autoimmune hyperthyroidism, sleep apnoea, and alcohol use disorders, AF/L demonstrated a causal association with POAG. However, studies on the relationship between AF/L and glaucoma are limited. Potential risk factors for cardiovascular disorders include systemic hypertension, hypotension, vasospasm, elevated blood viscosity, and diabetes, particularly in the absence of elevated IOP [45]. Considering that vascular dysfunction is one of the known mechanisms of glaucoma, AF/L may be considered a cause of glaucoma. According to a longitudinal study on the association between AF and risk of glaucoma [19], AF leads to an increased risk of glaucoma (hazard ratio = 1.31, 95% CI = 1.15–1.48) with variable adjustment. In the sequence of AF onset, conditions are amenable to the formation of an intracardiac thrombus or embolus [46]. According to the literature, AF/L remains one of the main contributors to stroke, unexpected death, and cardiovascular morbidity [13,47]. AF is independently linked to a 1.5-fold higher risk of all-cause mortality in men and a 2-fold higher risk in women [48]. In clinical ophthalmological practice, microembolic complications may remain unreported [49,50]. Reperfusion injury is caused by repeated microemboli occlusion of the central retinal artery, branched posterior ciliary artery, or ophthalmic artery at any level followed by reperfusion, resulting in unstable ocular perfusion of the retina or choroid [18]. Recurrent transient ischaemic episodes can cause retinal ganglion cell death and perfusion disruption, and subsequently glaucoma. Considering that migraine and orthostatic hypotension are risk factors for POAG [51], the presence of AF/L is potentially associated with POAG.

AF/L is characterised by a highly irregular heart rate, which may contribute to unstable ocular perfusion. Given that high IOP is the primary risk factor for POAG, researchers may be curious about the effects of AF/L on IOP as a mechanism of POAG. To address these concerns, the effect of AF/L on IOP through MR analysis indicated that there was no effect on IOP changes (Supplementary Tables S3–S5). These results support the vascular theory of POAG aetiology, and AF/L may cause POAG because of unstable perfusion pressure rather than IOP. Several studies have suggested a potential association between glaucoma and AF [17]. One study identified correlations between cardiac arrhythmias, particularly AF, with visual field abnormalities and a decline in visual acuity in older patients with glaucoma. AF was also significantly more common in patients with glaucoma than in control participants [52]. Another hospital-based study of Polish patients found that AF, independent of other established cardiovascular risk factors, was associated with an increased risk of normal-tension glaucoma [18]. Normal-tension glaucoma may be influenced by factors other than IOP; however, it is included in the POAG spectrum. Recently, a study using Korean National Health Insurance Service data determined via cross-sectional analysis showed that the AF group had higher incidence rates of diabetes, hypertension, glaucoma, and chronic nephropathy [19]. In addition, a longitudinal analysis showed that patients with AF had a significantly higher cumulative incidence of glaucoma at 11 years (4.37% in the control group vs. 6.42% in the AF group) [19]. In addition, a reduced retinal capillary plexus precedes retinal ganglion cell loss in ocular hypertension [53], and macular microvascular damage is highly associated with visual field defects in POAG [54]. Considering these studies and our results simultaneously, it can be concluded that AF/L and vascular dysregulation can independently cause POAG. Although the primary focus of this study was POAG, angle-closure glaucoma should be considered when interpreting the results. Nevertheless, because this study analysed a large dataset for the risk of glaucoma compared with the severity of AF, its results are expected to be meaningful if interpreted in comparison with the study results.

Hypertension has been suggested as a risk factor for glaucoma, with a higher incidence in patients with POAG (OR = 1.55, $p < 0.001$) [55]. In addition, a Cox regression study found that untreated hypertension led to a greater risk of POAG [56]. AF/L and systemic hypertension frequently coexist with AF because arterial hypertension increases the risk of developing new-onset AF, and because both conditions share common risk factors and underlying pathophysiological mechanisms that contribute to their incidence [57]. A recent MR study indicated that hyperthyroidism is associated with AF, reporting that a genetically elevated FT3:FT4 ratio and hyperthyroidism, rather than FT4 levels within the reference range, are associated with an increased risk of developing AF [58]. Additionally, one study reported that individuals with thyroid eye disease in the All-of-Us Research Program were significantly more likely to be diagnosed with glaucoma [59]. Sleep apnoea is associated with POAG [60], and obstructive sleep apnoea is considered a complex and dynamic substrate for AF [61,62]. Moreover, alcohol consumption is a common trigger for AF/L, especially habitual alcohol intake [63]. A meta-analysis suggested a harmful association between alcohol use and OAG, with IOP elevation [64]. These variables are relevant confounders in studies of the association between AF/L and glaucoma. However, incorporating additional covariates, such as hypertension, autoimmune hyperthyroidism, sleep apnoea, and alcohol use disorder, into our multivariable MR analysis did not alter the significant association between AF/L and POAG. This suggests that the observed relationship between AF/L and POAG was not confounded by these factors, further supporting the causality of the association.

The primary strength of our study lies in the use of a relatively large cohort dataset, which provided evidence suggesting a causal effect of AF/L on POAG. While the study provides robust evidence for a causal relationship between these conditions, it is essential to consider limitations such as the generalisability of the findings to non-European populations, as the dataset was predominantly derived from European cohorts (Finland and the UK). Further research is required to determine whether these results can be generalised to other ethnic groups. Additionally, potential residual confounding factors cannot be ruled out despite multivariable adjustments. This study lacked access to individual-level data, which limited our ability to account for various confounding factors because our analysis relied on summary statistics derived from two-sample MR methods. We were also unable to assess the potential interactions between AF/L and other risk factors, such as hypertension, diabetes, or sleep apnoea, owing to the aggregated nature of the GWAS summary statistics used in our study. Future studies with access to individual-level data are warranted to explore these interactions and their impact on causal pathways. However, the methods employed to validate the MR hypotheses did not provide absolute confirmation. Violations of underlying MR assumptions may lead to erroneous conclusions, necessitating a cautious interpretation of the findings. The conditional F-statistics for the confounders included in the multivariable MR analysis were below the conventional threshold of 10 ($F = 4.08$ for autoimmune hyperthyroidism; $F = 3.19$ for sleep apnoea; and $F = 3.21$ for alcohol use disorder), indicating the presence of potentially weak instruments. To address this issue, we performed an IVW analysis with Q-minimisation (Q-het), which is robust against weak instruments and heterogeneity, to validate our findings. Even with the application of robust methods, the non-significant results for certain confounders require cautious interpretation as they may reflect limited statistical power due to weak instruments. Finally, because the prevalence rates of AF/L and POAG were not high (2% and 3%, respectively), GWAS of rare diseases using biobank data may face a severe imbalance in the number of cases and controls [65], which may produce false-positive GWAS hits [66]. When these hits are selected as IVs, they can bias the MR estimates. However, the GWAS summary statistics used in this study employed methods designed to address case-control imbalances, such as SAIGE and the firth test [65,67]. These approaches have been shown to efficiently control false-positive associations and enhance the reliability of selected IVs. Future studies could benefit from the inclusion of larger and more diverse cohorts, as well as the investigation of the specific pathways through which AF/L influences POAG risk.

5. Conclusions

The findings contribute to the understanding of the relationship between AF/L and POAG and suggest that AF/L may increase the risk of POAG. This has potential clinical implications as it highlights the importance of monitoring glaucoma risk in patients with AF/L. In addition, the value of this study lies in the recommendation that, in cases where AF/L is diagnosed in a clinical setting, ophthalmological screening should be advised to monitor the development of glaucoma. Conversely, when glaucoma is diagnosed, AF/L should be included in the medical history questionnaire for further evaluation. Further research should explore the biological mechanisms underlying this association and determine whether the effective management of AF/L could reduce the incidence of POAG.

Supplementary Materials: The following supporting information can be downloaded at https://www.mdpi.com/article/10.3390/jcm13247670/s1. Table S1: List of SNPs used as IVs in univariate MR analysis; Table S2: Multivariate MR-IVW analysis with minimised Q statistics; Table S3: Summary of intraocular pressure data; Table S4: Univariate MR results of the causal effects of AF/L on intraocular pressure; Table S5: Multivariable MR results of the causal effects of AF/L on intraocular pressure.

Author Contributions: J.H.S. and Y.L. designed the study and collected the data, Y.L. performed the statistical analysis, and J.H.S. drafted the manuscript. All authors have reviewed and edited the previous versions of the manuscript. All authors have read and agreed to the published version of the manuscript.

Funding: This study was supported by a National Research Foundation of Korea (NRF) grant funded by the Korean Government (Ministry of Science and ICT) (no. 2022R1C1C1002929) and a Veterans Health Service Medical Centre research grant (no. VHSMC24002). The funders had no role in the study design, collection, analyses, interpretation of data, writing of the manuscript, or decision to publish the results.

Institutional Review Board Statement: This study was conducted in accordance with the tenets of the Declaration of Helsinki and approved by the Institutional Review Board of the Veterans Health Service Medical Centre (no. 2023-12-030, approved on 11 January 2024).

Informed Consent Statement: Informed consent was not required because anonymised and deidentified data were used in the analyses. The requirement for patient consent was waived because of the retrospective nature of the study.

Data Availability Statement: The datasets used and/or analysed in the current study are available from FinnGen (https://finngen.gitbook.io/documentation/data-download, accessed on 4 November 2023) and the GWAS catalogue (https://www.ebi.ac.uk/gwas/summary-statistics, accessed on 4 November 2023).

Acknowledgments: We would like to thank FinnGen (https://www.finngen.fi/en) and the GWAS catalogue (https://www.ebi.ac.uk/gwas).

Conflicts of Interest: The authors declare no conflicts of interest. The funders had no role in the study design; collection, analyses, or interpretation of data; writing of the manuscript; or decision to publish the results.

References

1. Weinreb, R.N.; Aung, T.; Medeiros, F.A. The pathophysiology and treatment of glaucoma: A review. *JAMA* **2014**, *311*, 1901–1911. [CrossRef] [PubMed]
2. Li, T.; Lindsley, K.; Rouse, B.; Hong, H.; Shi, Q.; Friedman, D.S.; Wormald, R.; Dickersin, K. Comparative Effectiveness of First-Line Medications for Primary Open-Angle Glaucoma: A Systematic Review and Network Meta-analysis. *Ophthalmology* **2016**, *123*, 129–140. [CrossRef] [PubMed]
3. Luo, L.J.; Nguyen, D.D.; Lai, J.Y. Benzoic acid derivative-modified chitosan-g-poly(N-isopropylacrylamide): Methoxylation effects and pharmacological treatments of Glaucoma-related neurodegeneration. *J. Control Release* **2020**, *317*, 246–258. [CrossRef] [PubMed]
4. Jonas, J.B.; Aung, T.; Bourne, R.R.; Bron, A.M.; Ritch, R.; Panda-Jonas, S. Glaucoma. *Lancet* **2017**, *390*, 2183–2193. [CrossRef] [PubMed]
5. Shin, H.T.; Yoon, B.W.; Seo, J.H. Analysis of risk allele frequencies of single nucleotide polymorphisms related to open-angle glaucoma in different ethnic groups. *BMC Med. Genom.* **2021**, *14*, 80. [CrossRef]
6. Seo, J.H.; Kim, T.W.; Weinreb, R.N. Lamina cribrosa depth in healthy eyes. *Investig. Ophthalmol. Vis. Sci.* **2014**, *55*, 1241–1251. [CrossRef]
7. Yanagi, M.; Kawasaki, R.; Wang, J.J.; Wong, T.Y.; Crowston, J.; Kiuchi, Y. Vascular risk factors in glaucoma: A review. *Clin. Exp. Ophthalmol.* **2011**, *39*, 252–258. [CrossRef]
8. Jonas, J.B. Role of cerebrospinal fluid pressure in the pathogenesis of glaucoma. *Acta Ophthalmol.* **2011**, *89*, 505–514. [CrossRef]
9. Seo, J.H.; Kim, T.W.; Weinreb, R.N.; Kim, Y.A.; Kim, M. Relationship of intraocular pressure and frequency of spontaneous retinal venous pulsation in primary open-angle glaucoma. *Ophthalmology* **2012**, *119*, 2254–2260. [CrossRef]
10. Flammer, J.; Mozaffarieh, M. What is the present pathogenetic concept of glaucomatous optic neuropathy? *Surv. Ophthalmol.* **2007**, *52* (Suppl. S2), S162–S173. [CrossRef]
11. Wierzbowska, J.; Wierzbowski, R.; Stankiewicz, A.; Siesky, B.; Harris, A. Cardiac autonomic dysfunction in patients with normal tension glaucoma: 24-h heart rate and blood pressure variability analysis. *Br. J. Ophthalmol.* **2012**, *96*, 624–628. [CrossRef] [PubMed]
12. Li, X.; Liu, Z.; Jiang, X.; Xia, R.; Li, Y.; Pan, X.; Yao, Y.; Fan, X. Global, regional, and national burdens of atrial fibrillation/flutter from 1990 to 2019: An age-period-cohort analysis using the Global Burden of Disease 2019 study. *J. Glob. Health* **2023**, *13*, 04154. [CrossRef] [PubMed]
13. Elsheikh, S.; Hill, A.; Irving, G.; Lip, G.Y.H.; Abdul-Rahim, A.H. Atrial fibrillation and stroke: State-of-the-art and future directions. *Curr. Probl. Cardiol.* **2024**, *49*, 102181. [CrossRef] [PubMed]
14. Mareedu, R.K.; Abdalrahman, I.B.; Dharmashankar, K.C.; Granada, J.F.; Chyou, P.H.; Sharma, P.P.; Smith, P.N.; Hayes, J.J.; Greenlee, R.T.; Vidaillet, H. Atrial flutter versus atrial fibrillation in a general population: Differences in comorbidities associated with their respective onset. *Clin. Med. Res.* **2010**, *8*, 1–6. [CrossRef]
15. Waldo, A.L.; Feld, G.K. Inter-relationships of atrial fibrillation and atrial flutter mechanisms and clinical implications. *J. Am. Coll. Cardiol.* **2008**, *51*, 779–786. [CrossRef]
16. Bikbov, M.M.; Kazakbaeva, G.M.; Rakhimova, E.M.; Panda-Jonas, S.; Fakhretdinova, A.A.; Tuliakova, A.M.; Rusakova, I.A.; Jonas, J.B. Atrial fibrillation and flutter and ocular diseases. The Ural eye and medical study and the Ural very old study. *Acta Ophthalmol.* **2024**, *102*, e1057–e1065. [CrossRef]
17. Flammer, J.; Orgul, S.; Costa, V.P.; Orzalesi, N.; Krieglstein, G.K.; Serra, L.M.; Renard, J.P.; Stefansson, E. The impact of ocular blood flow in glaucoma. *Prog. Retin. Eye Res.* **2002**, *21*, 359–393. [CrossRef]
18. Zaleska-Zmijewska, A.; Janiszewski, M.; Wawrzyniak, Z.M.; Kuch, M.; Szaflik, J.; Szaflik, J.P. Is atrial fibrillation a risk factor for normal-tension glaucoma? *Medicine* **2017**, *96*, e8347. [CrossRef]
19. Cho, H.K.; Han, J.C.; Choi, J.A.; Chae, J.E.; Kim, R.B. Association between atrial fibrillation and the risk of glaucoma development: A 12-year Nationwide cohort study. *Eye* **2023**, *37*, 2033–2041. [CrossRef]
20. Burgess, S.; Thompson, S.G. Multivariable Mendelian randomization: The use of pleiotropic genetic variants to estimate causal effects. *Am. J. Epidemiol.* **2015**, *181*, 251–260. [CrossRef]
21. Burgess, S.; Thompson, S.G. Interpreting findings from Mendelian randomization using the MR-Egger method. *Eur. J. Epidemiol.* **2017**, *32*, 377–389. [CrossRef]
22. Seo, J.H.; Lee, Y. Possible Causal Association between Type 2 Diabetes and Glycaemic Traits in Primary Open-Angle Glaucoma: A Two-Sample Mendelian Randomisation Study. *Biomedicines* **2024**, *12*, 866. [CrossRef]
23. Wang, K.; Yang, F.; Liu, X.; Lin, X.; Yin, H.; Tang, Q.; Jiang, L.; Yao, K. Appraising the Effects of Metabolic Traits on the Risk of Glaucoma: A Mendelian Randomization Study. *Metabolites* **2023**, *13*, 109. [CrossRef]
24. Chong, R.S.; Li, H.; Cheong, A.J.Y.; Fan, Q.; Koh, V.; Raghavan, L.; Nongpiur, M.E.; Cheng, C.Y. Mendelian Randomization Implicates Bidirectional Association between Myopia and Primary Open-Angle Glaucoma or Intraocular Pressure. *Ophthalmology* **2023**, *130*, 394–403. [CrossRef]
25. Sakaue, S.; Kanai, M.; Tanigawa, Y.; Karjalainen, J.; Kurki, M.; Koshiba, S.; Narita, A.; Konuma, T.; Yamamoto, K.; Akiyama, M.; et al. A cross-population atlas of genetic associations for 220 human phenotypes. *Nat. Genet.* **2021**, *53*, 1415–1424. [CrossRef]

26. Choquet, H.; Paylakhi, S.; Kneeland, S.C.; Thai, K.K.; Hoffmann, T.J.; Yin, J.; Kvale, M.N.; Banda, Y.; Tolman, N.G.; Williams, P.A.; et al. A multiethnic genome-wide association study of primary open-angle glaucoma identifies novel risk loci. *Nat. Commun.* **2018**, *9*, 2278. [CrossRef]
27. Kurki, M.I.; Karjalainen, J.; Palta, P.; Sipila, T.P.; Kristiansson, K.; Donner, K.M.; Reeve, M.P.; Laivuori, H.; Aavikko, M.; Kaunisto, M.A.; et al. FinnGen provides genetic insights from a well-phenotyped isolated population. *Nature* **2023**, *613*, 508–518. [CrossRef]
28. Jiang, L.; Zheng, Z.; Fang, H.; Yang, J. A generalized linear mixed model association tool for biobank-scale data. *Nat. Genet.* **2021**, *53*, 1616–1621. [CrossRef]
29. Burgess, S.; Thompson, S.G.; CRP CHD Genetics Collaboration. Avoiding bias from weak instruments in Mendelian randomization studies. *Int. J. Epidemiol.* **2011**, *40*, 755–764. [CrossRef]
30. Burgess, S.; Butterworth, A.; Thompson, S.G. Mendelian randomization analysis with multiple genetic variants using summarized data. *Genet. Epidemiol.* **2013**, *37*, 658–665. [CrossRef]
31. Sanderson, E.; Spiller, W.; Bowden, J. Testing and correcting for weak and pleiotropic instruments in two-sample multivariable Mendelian randomization. *Stat. Med.* **2021**, *40*, 5434–5452. [CrossRef]
32. Bowden, J.; Del Greco, M.F.; Minelli, C.; Davey Smith, G.; Sheehan, N.; Thompson, J. A framework for the investigation of pleiotropy in two-sample summary data Mendelian randomization. *Stat. Med.* **2017**, *36*, 1783–1802. [CrossRef]
33. Lee, Y.; Kim, Y.A.; Seo, J.H. Causal Association of Obesity and Dyslipidemia with Type 2 Diabetes: A Two-Sample Mendelian Randomization Study. *Genes* **2022**, *13*, 2407. [CrossRef]
34. Burgess, S.; Davey Smith, G.; Davies, N.M.; Dudbridge, F.; Gill, D.; Glymour, M.M.; Hartwig, F.P.; Holmes, M.V.; Minelli, C.; Relton, C.L.; et al. Guidelines for performing Mendelian randomization investigations. *Wellcome Open Res.* **2019**, *4*, 186. [CrossRef]
35. Bowden, J.; Davey Smith, G.; Haycock, P.C.; Burgess, S. Consistent Estimation in Mendelian Randomization with Some Invalid Instruments Using a Weighted Median Estimator. *Genet. Epidemiol.* **2016**, *40*, 304–314. [CrossRef]
36. Bowden, J.; Davey Smith, G.; Burgess, S. Mendelian randomization with invalid instruments: Effect estimation and bias detection through Egger regression. *Int. J. Epidemiol.* **2015**, *44*, 512–525. [CrossRef]
37. Bowden, J.; Del Greco, M.F.; Minelli, C.; Davey Smith, G.; Sheehan, N.A.; Thompson, J.R. Assessing the suitability of summary data for two-sample Mendelian randomization analyses using MR-Egger regression: The role of the I2 statistic. *Int. J. Epidemiol.* **2016**, *45*, 1961–1974. [CrossRef]
38. Greco, M.F.; Minelli, C.; Sheehan, N.A.; Thompson, J.R. Detecting pleiotropy in Mendelian randomisation studies with summary data and a continuous outcome. *Stat. Med.* **2015**, *34*, 2926–2940. [CrossRef]
39. Verbanck, M.; Chen, C.Y.; Neale, B.; Do, R. Publisher Correction: Detection of widespread horizontal pleiotropy in causal relationships inferred from Mendelian randomization between complex traits and diseases. *Nat. Genet.* **2018**, *50*, 1196. [CrossRef]
40. Rees, J.M.B.; Wood, A.M.; Burgess, S. Extending the MR-Egger method for multivariable Mendelian randomization to correct for both measured and unmeasured pleiotropy. *Stat. Med.* **2017**, *36*, 4705–4718. [CrossRef]
41. Bulik-Sullivan, B.K.; Loh, P.R.; Finucane, H.K.; Ripke, S.; Yang, J.; Patterson, N.; Daly, M.J.; Price, A.L.; Neale, B.M.; Schizophrenia Working Group of the Psychiatric Genomics Consortium. Score regression distinguishes confounding from polygenicity in genome-wide association studies. *Nat. Genet.* **2015**, *47*, 291–295. [CrossRef] [PubMed]
42. Bulik-Sullivan, B.; Finucane, H.K.; Anttila, V.; Gusev, A.; Day, F.R.; Loh, P.R.; ReproGen, C.; Psychiatric Genomics Consortium; Duncan, L.; Genetic Consortium for Anorexia Nervosa of the Wellcome Trust Case Control Consortium; et al. An atlas of genetic correlations across human diseases and traits. *Nat. Genet.* **2015**, *47*, 1236–1241. [CrossRef]
43. Zheng, J.; Richardson, T.G.; Millard, L.A.C.; Hemani, G.; Elsworth, B.L.; Raistrick, C.A.; Vilhjalmsson, B.; Neale, B.M.; Haycock, P.C.; Smith, G.D.; et al. PhenoSpD: An integrated toolkit for phenotypic correlation estimation and multiple testing correction using GWAS summary statistics. *Gigascience* **2018**, *7*, giy090. [CrossRef]
44. Jin, H.; Lee, S.; Won, S. Causal Evaluation of Laboratory Markers in Type 2 Diabetes on Cancer and Vascular Diseases Using Various Mendelian Randomization Tools. *Front. Genet.* **2020**, *11*, 597420. [CrossRef]
45. Broadway, D.C.; Drance, S.M. Glaucoma and vasospasm. *Br. J. Ophthalmol.* **1998**, *82*, 862–870. [CrossRef]
46. Migdady, I.; Russman, A.; Buletko, A.B. Atrial Fibrillation and Ischemic Stroke: A Clinical Review. *Semin. Neurol.* **2021**, *41*, 348–364. [CrossRef]
47. Naser, N.; Kulic, M.; Dilic, M.; Dzubur, A.; Durak, A.; Pepic, E.; Smajic, E.; Kusljugic, Z. The Cumulative Incidence of Stroke, Myocardial infarction, Heart Failure and Sudden Cardiac Death in Patients with Atrial Fibrillation. *Med. Arch.* **2017**, *71*, 316–319. [CrossRef]
48. Lip, G.Y.H.; Proietti, M.; Potpara, T.; Mansour, M.; Savelieva, I.; Tse, H.F.; Goette, A.; Camm, A.J.; Blomstrom-Lundqvist, C.; Gupta, D.; et al. Atrial fibrillation and stroke prevention: 25 years of research at EP Europace journal. *Europace* **2023**, *25*, euad226. [CrossRef]
49. Hayreh, S.S.; Podhajsky, P.A.; Zimmerman, M.B. Retinal artery occlusion: Associated systemic and ophthalmic abnormalities. *Ophthalmology* **2009**, *116*, 1928–1936. [CrossRef]
50. Yen, J.C.; Lin, H.L.; Hsu, C.A.; Li, Y.C.; Hsu, M.H. Atrial Fibrillation and Coronary Artery Disease as Risk Factors of Retinal Artery Occlusion: A Nationwide Population-Based Study. *BioMed Res. Int.* **2015**, *2015*, 374616. [CrossRef]
51. Flammer, J.; Konieczka, K.; Flammer, A.J. The primary vascular dysregulation syndrome: Implications for eye diseases. *EPMA J.* **2013**, *4*, 14. [CrossRef] [PubMed]

52. Perasalo, R.; Perasalo, J.; Raitta, C. Electrocardiographic changes in institutionalized geriatric glaucoma patients. *Graefes Arch. Clin. Exp. Ophthalmol.* **1992**, *230*, 213–217. [CrossRef] [PubMed]
53. Pitale, P.M.; Shen, G.; Sigireddi, R.R.; Polo-Prieto, M.; Park, Y.H.; Gibson, S.E.; Westenskow, P.D.; Channa, R.; Frankfort, B.J. Selective vulnerability of the intermediate retinal capillary plexus precedes retinal ganglion cell loss in ocular hypertension. *Front. Cell Neurosci.* **2022**, *16*, 1073786. [CrossRef] [PubMed]
54. Tao, A.; Liang, Y.; Chen, J.; Hu, H.; Huang, Q.; Zheng, J.; Ye, C.; Lu, F. Structure-function correlation of localized visual field defects and macular microvascular damage in primary open-angle glaucoma. *Microvasc. Res.* **2020**, *130*, 104005. [CrossRef]
55. Wu, J.; Wang, H.; Yu, S. Hypertension as a Risk Factor for Primary Open-angle Glaucoma: A Meta-analysis. *J. Coll. Physicians Surg. Pak.* **2023**, *33*, 915–918. [CrossRef]
56. Lee, J.S.; Kim, Y.J.; Kim, S.; Bae, H.W.; Kim, S.S.; Lee, S.W.; Kim, C.Y. Increased Risks of Open-Angle Glaucoma in Untreated Hypertension. *Am. J. Ophthalmol.* **2023**, *252*, 111–120. [CrossRef]
57. Kallistratos, M.S.; Poulimenos, L.E.; Manolis, A.J. Atrial fibrillation and arterial hypertension. *Pharmacol. Res.* **2018**, *128*, 322–326. [CrossRef]
58. Ellervik, C.; Roselli, C.; Christophersen, I.E.; Alonso, A.; Pietzner, M.; Sitlani, C.M.; Trompet, S.; Arking, D.E.; Geelhoed, B.; Guo, X.; et al. Assessment of the Relationship Between Genetic Determinants of Thyroid Function and Atrial Fibrillation: A Mendelian Randomization Study. *JAMA Cardiol.* **2019**, *4*, 144–152. [CrossRef]
59. Delavar, A.; Saseendrakumar, B.R.; Lee, T.C. Associations Between Thyroid Eye Disease and Glaucoma Among Those Enrolled in the National Institutes of Health All of Us Research Program: Corrigendum. *Ophthalmic Plast. Reconstr. Surg.* **2023**, *39*, 405. [CrossRef]
60. Leggewie, B.; Gouveris, H.; Bahr, K. A Narrative Review of the Association between Obstructive Sleep Apnea and Glaucoma in Adults. *Int. J. Mol. Sci.* **2022**, *23*, 10080. [CrossRef]
61. Linz, D.; Nattel, S.; Kalman, J.M.; Sanders, P. Sleep Apnea and Atrial Fibrillation. *Card. Electrophysiol. Clin.* **2021**, *13*, 87–94. [CrossRef] [PubMed]
62. Chung, M.K.; Eckhardt, L.L.; Chen, L.Y.; Ahmed, H.M.; Gopinathannair, R.; Joglar, J.A.; Noseworthy, P.A.; Pack, Q.R.; Sanders, P.; Trulock, K.M.; et al. Lifestyle and Risk Factor Modification for Reduction of Atrial Fibrillation: A Scientific Statement From the American Heart Association. *Circulation* **2020**, *141*, e750–e772. [CrossRef] [PubMed]
63. Voskoboinik, A.; Marcus, G.M. The Impact of Alcohol Intake on Atrial Fibrillation. *Curr. Cardiol. Rep.* **2020**, *22*, 111. [CrossRef] [PubMed]
64. Stuart, K.V.; Madjedi, K.; Luben, R.N.; Chua, S.Y.L.; Warwick, A.N.; Chia, M.; Pasquale, L.R.; Wiggs, J.L.; Kang, J.H.; Hysi, P.G.; et al. Alcohol, Intraocular Pressure, and Open-Angle Glaucoma: A Systematic Review and Meta-analysis. *Ophthalmology* **2022**, *129*, 637–652. [CrossRef]
65. Zhou, W.; Nielsen, J.B.; Fritsche, L.G.; Dey, R.; Gabrielsen, M.E.; Wolford, B.N.; LeFaive, J.; VandeHaar, P.; Gagliano, S.A.; Gifford, A.; et al. Efficiently controlling for case-control imbalance and sample relatedness in large-scale genetic association studies. *Nat. Genet.* **2018**, *50*, 1335–1341. [CrossRef]
66. Zhao, S.S.; Burgess, S. Use of Mendelian randomization to assess the causal status of modifiable exposures for rheumatic diseases. *Best Pract. Res. Clin. Rheumatol.* **2024**, *38*, 101967. [CrossRef]
67. Wang, X. Firth logistic regression for rare variant association tests. *Front. Genet.* **2014**, *5*, 187. [CrossRef]

Journal of
Clinical Medicine

MDPI

Article

Five-Year Outcomes of Deep Sclerectomy in Pseudoexfoliation Glaucoma Compared to Primary Open-Angle Glaucoma

Carlo Fiore [1,*], Xiao Shang [1,2], Joel-Benjamin Lincke [1], Nathanael Urs Häner [1], Martin Sebastian Zinkernagel [1] and Jan Darius Unterlauft [1,*]

1 Department of Ophthalmology, Inselspital, Bern University Hospital, University of Bern, Freiburgstrasse 18, 3010 Bern, Switzerland

2 Graduate School for Cellular and Biomedical Sciences, University of Bern, Mittelstrasse 43, 3012 Bern, Switzerland

* Correspondence: carlo.fiore@students.unibe.ch (C.F.); jandarius.unterlauft@insel.ch (J.D.U.)

Abstract: Objectives: This study aimed to investigate the five-year outcomes of deep sclerectomy (DS) in patients with pseudoexfoliation glaucoma (PEXG) and primary open-angle glaucoma (POAG). **Methods**: This retrospective, observational, unicentric study analyzed POAG and PEXG patients. Intraocular pressure (IOP), the number of IOP-lowering medications, peripapillary retinal nerve fiber layer (RNFL) thickness, the number of postoperative interventions, surgical success rates, and secondary surgery rates were evaluated at baseline and during follow-up appointments. **Results**: A total of 109 POAG and 153 PEXG eyes were included. Over the 5-year follow-up, IOP decreased in both groups ($p = 0.17$), from 22.8 ± 0.7 to 13.3 ± 0.6 mmHg ($p < 0.001$; POAG) and from 24.3 ± 0.8 to 16.6 ± 1.2 mmHg ($p < 0.001$; PEXG). The number of IOP-lowering medications decreased comparably ($p = 0.99$), from 3.1 ± 0.1 to 1.7 ± 0.3 ($p = 0.001$; POAG) and from 3.4 ± 0.1 to 1.7 ± 0.2 ($p < 0.001$; PEXG). Peripapillary RNFL thickness decreased in both groups ($p = 0.31$), from 60.6 ± 1.9 to 54.2 ± 2.4 μm ($p < 0.001$; POAG) and from 63.1 ± 1.7 to 58.0 ± 2.3 μm ($p < 0.001$; PEXG). The 5-year complete success rates were 33% and 12% for the POAG and PEXG groups, respectively ($p = 0.01$). The qualified success rates were 63% and 40% ($p = 0.03$). Secondary glaucoma surgery was required in 8% of POAG eyes and 21% of PEXG eyes ($p = 0.04$). **Conclusions**: DS resulted in comparable results for IOP, medications, and RNFL development in the PEXG and POAG groups but in less favorable outcomes concerning surgical success and further necessary repeated glaucoma surgery in patients with PEXG over the 5-year follow-up period.

Keywords: glaucoma; deep sclerectomy; primary open-angle glaucoma; pseudoexfoliation glaucoma; glaucoma surgery outcomes; retinal nerve fiber layer

1. Introduction

Glaucoma is a cluster of medical conditions with diverse pathophysiological processes, sharing progressive optic disc cupping with retinal ganglion cell loss and consequent visual field defects [1]. These changes are strongly related but apparently not exclusively due to intraocular pressure (IOP) [2]. Primary open-angle glaucoma (POAG) is characterized by an open anterior chamber angle without any secondary disease etiology and is the most frequent type of glaucoma in Europe and Northern America, with a prevalence in people aged 40–80 years of 2.51% and 3.29%, respectively [3,4]. Pseudoexfoliation glaucoma (PEXG) is due to pseudoexfoliation syndrome (PEX), a systemic disorder that leads to abnormal deposits composed predominantly of fibrillary material [5]. The prevalence of PEX has been reported to vary widely between regions, ranging from 4% to 21% in different European countries [6]. These deposits can result in the degeneration of Schlemm's canal and aqueous humor outflow obstruction in the trabecular meshwork, increasing IOP and inducing glaucoma [7]. A number of topical and systemic medications, as well as laser and surgical procedures, can help reduce IOP [8], which as of today, is the only proven effective treatment to decelerate or, at best, stop disease progression [2]. Usually, conservative approaches are preferred initially. Though multiple classes of medications exist, failure to meet IOP targets and disease progression despite maximally tolerated conservative treatment can indicate the need for interventional surgical therapy [8].

One of the first choices is trabeculectomy (TE) [9], a technique which functions through the creation of a direct transscleral fistula for the aqueous humor to reach the subconjunctival space [10]. This approach has been observed to be prone to complications [11], leading to the search for less invasive and safer techniques leading to similar results. Deep sclerectomy (DS) is a surgical procedure developed with this intent. It increases aqueous humor outflow from the anterior chamber into the subconjunctival space under a scleral flap [12]. Its aim is to provide substantial IOP reduction with fewer complications than TE [13].

PEXG is associated with faster progression compared to POAG [14]. The amount of deposited pseudoexfoliation material in the aqueous humor outflow system has been observed to be related to disease severity [15]. Considering this and the pathomechanism behind PEXG, non-penetrating filtering surgery such as DS may not be the perfect option in the long term, since the trabecular meshwork is left in place and congestion by pseudoexfoliation material is proceeding. As of today, DS has only been observed to be effective for PEXG patients in trials that either had smaller groups, shorter observation times, or both compared to our herein presented study [16–22].

The aim of this study was to investigate the five-year outcomes of DS for PEXG compared to POAG cases. This information could help provide targeted surgical care for these patient populations. Therefore, we retrospectively investigated the course of functional and anatomical parameters, as well as the development of complete and qualified success rates, in a comparative group of POAG and PEXG cases followed-up over the first 5 years after surgery.

2. Materials and Methods

This retrospective, observational, unicentric study is a sub-analysis of previously collected data from the Bern Glaucoma Registry Study (BGRS). The BGRS is a retrospective medical records review study conducted at the Department of Ophthalmology, Inselspital, Bern University Hospital. Consecutive medical records of patients over 18 years old who underwent glaucoma surgery between 2012 and 2023 were reviewed for eligibility. The BGRS was approved by the Ethics Committee of the Canton of Bern (BASEC-ID: 2022-01046) and adhered to the tenets of the Declaration of Helsinki. Informed consent for participants was waived due to the retrospective nature of this study.

Patients diagnosed with POAG or PEXG who underwent DS between July 2012 and November 2023 were included. The minimum sample size required to detect a 20% difference in surgical success rates (expected to lie at 60% and 40% for complete and qualified success for each group, respectively) with a 95% confidence interval and power of 0.80 was calculated to be 107 eyes for each cohort. Indications for glaucoma surgery were disease progression, above-target IOP on maximum tolerable medical therapy, or the inability to escalate medical therapy further due to existing allergies or other medical conditions. Disease progression was defined as a worsening of the visual field mean defect (MD) on three consecutive tests with an increase of at least −2.00 dB within one year. The decision to perform DS and not any of the other available surgical options was usually made at the discretion of the treating physician during outpatient examination. Medical records were reviewed, and clinical data were added to the BGRS database and subsequently analyzed. Eyes/patients with co-existing ocular or central nervous system diseases that could affect the ophthalmic tests performed (i.e., excessive myopia, macular degeneration, multiple sclerosis, etc.) were excluded. If both eyes of a single patient were eligible, only the first eye undergoing surgery was included to reduce the effect of data compounding due to bilateral eyes [23].

2.1. Surgical Procedures

Surgeries were performed by 4 experienced ophthalmic surgeons following standard surgical procedures described in previous studies [24,25]. The minimum and maximum number of years of experience with which a surgeon operated on the patients in the study was 7 and 20 years, respectively. These were defined as the time between their first year as an attending surgeon and the first or last year in which they operated on the patients included in the study. In summary, a fornix-based conjunctival flap was created. Mitomycin C (0.2 mg/mL) was applied for 2 min and meticulously rinsed thereafter with balanced salt solution. A 5 × 5 mm scleral flap was dissected, and another 2 × 2 mm deeper flap was excised to gain access to Schlemm's canal and expose the trabeculo-Descemet window. The scleral flap was then re-approximated with two non-absorbable 10/0 interrupted sutures that were adapted according to resulting IOP. An ocular viscoelastic device (OVD) was injected beneath the scleral flap to prevent its collapse onto the scleral bed. Tenon's capsule and conjunctiva were re-approximated to the limbus with two to four absorbable interrupted sutures. Non-absorbable mattress sutures were used to guarantee water tightness and left in situ for three weeks postoperatively. The postoperative medical plan consisted of topical tobramycin four times a day for three weeks and atropine at 0.5% twice a day for one week or equivalents. Topical prednisolone acetate or equivalent was administered four times a day for three weeks and subsequently tapered according to clinical evaluation. The follow-up plan usually included weekly examinations during the first postoperative month, with subsequent visits at 3 and 6 months and annually until 5 years postoperatively. Indications for corrective procedures were determined by the treating physician after an assessment of clinical presentation, disease course, and the resulting IOP.

2.2. Follow-Up Treatments and Data Collection

Data were collected from the hospital's electronic medical records in the documentation system FIDUS (version 21.42.2, Arztservice Wente GmbH, Darmstadt, Germany). Outcomes for each case were assessed preoperatively and at the following postoperative timepoints: 1 day, 1 month, 3 months, 6 months, 1 year, 2 years, 3 years, and 5 years. Not every case was examined at each timepoint. Collected data included the diagnosis of either POAG or PEXG, patient age at surgery, sex, laterality of the treated eye, history of previous glaucoma surgeries, IOP measurements, the number of IOP-lowering medications, best corrected visual acuity (BCVA), visual field MD, peripapillary retinal nerve fiber layer (RNFL) thickness, postoperative interventions, and secondary major glaucoma surgeries after DS. IOP was measured using Goldmann applanation tonometry (Haag-Streit, Köniz, Switzerland). Both topical and systemic IOP-lowering medications were documented. For combination drugs, each active ingredient was documented as a separate medication. BCVA was measured with Snellen charts and values were converted into logMAR units. The MD of visual field tests were assessed with standard automated perimetry (SAP) using Octopus 900 (Haag-Streit, Köniz, Switzerland). Peripapillary RNFL thickness was evaluated by spectral domain optical coherence tomography (OCT) using the Spectralis OCT machine (Heidelberg Engineering, Heidelberg, Germany). Postoperative interventions included iridoplasties, bleb needlings, Nd:YAG-laser goniopunctures, 5-fluorouracil (5-FU) injections (0.1 mL subconjunctival, 50 mg/mL), and open surgical revisions. Secondary major glaucoma surgeries were defined as subsequent interventions performed to alter glaucoma progression or symptoms. These were not directly related to the management of consequences resulting from the original DS and included the following procedures: cyclophotocoagulation, evisceration, TE, insertion of a Baerveldt Glaucoma Implant, PreserFlo MicroShunt, and XEN Gel Stent. Cataract surgeries were not included in this category of procedures. Subsequent interventions, including secondary major glaucoma surgeries, were performed after thorough examination by a specialized glaucoma surgeon, deciding on the necessity for an additional surgical intervention. Resulting IOP, the number of given IOP-lowering medication hinting towards surgical failure of DS, and further functional worsening in SAP were taken into account, leading to the decision for additional glaucoma surgery (usually trabeculectomy or cyclophotocoagulation).

Surgical success was evaluated at 1, 3, and 5 years after DS surgery. Qualified success had to meet each of the following three criteria: IOP reduction equal to or greater than 20% from preoperative values, a resulting IOP lower than 21 mmHg, and no secondary major glaucoma surgery performed from the time of the DS until the evaluated timepoint. Complete success had to meet each of the three aforementioned criteria without the application of additional IOP-lowering medication.

2.3. Data Analysis

Clinical data were gathered and plotted using the spreadsheet applications Microsoft Excel (Version 16.83, Microsoft Corporation, Redmond, WA, USA) and Numbers (Version 13.0, Apple Inc., Cupertino, CA, USA). The software IBM SPSS Statistics (Version 29.0.2.0, IBM, Armonk, NY, USA) was used to perform the statistical analysis and to plot clinical data. Continuous variables were expressed as mean values and standard error of the mean. Categorical variables were expressed as percentages. The data were collected and analyzed by one of the operating surgeons (J.D.U.) together with a medical student (C.F.).

The primary outcomes were changes in IOP, the number of IOP-lowering medications, the number of postoperative interventions, complete and qualified surgical success rates, and the number of secondary glaucoma surgeries over the course of 5 years after surgery. Secondary outcomes were BCVA, the MD, and peripapillary RNFL thickness at each timepoint. The following statistical tests were conducted: the chi-square test to compare categorical variables, the Wilcoxon signed-rank test to compare continuous non-parametric paired variables between different timepoints in the same group, the Mann–Whitney U test to compare continuous non-parametric unpaired variables at same timepoints between groups, and the two-tailed test for the Pearson and point biserial correlation coefficients. A p value less than 0.05 was considered statistically significant and is shown bolded in the tables.

3. Results

A total of 262 eyes (109 POAG eyes, 153 PEXG eyes) that underwent DS were included in the final analysis. Baseline demographic and clinical characteristics are shown in Table 1. The POAG group was younger than the PEXG group in this study (68.8 ± 1.0 years vs. 74.2 ± 0.6 years, $p < 0.001$). There was no statistically significant difference in laterality ($p = 0.23$) and the percentage of eyes with previous glaucoma surgery ($p = 0.67$). Differences in the mean IOP (mmHg), the number of IOP-lowering medications, BCVA (logMAR), visual field MD (dB), and RNFL thickness (µm) were not statistically significant between the POAG and PEXG groups. In the POAG cohort, two TEs and one DS were performed before the DS was analyzed. In contrast, three TEs were performed prior to DS in the PEXG cohort. The percentage of males was 56% in the POAG group and 36% in the PEXG group, and a statistically significant difference was present ($p = 0.001$).

Table 1. Baseline demographic and clinical characteristics of the study participants.

	POAG (n = 109)	**PEXG (n = 153)**	p
Age, yrs	68.8 ± 1.0	74.2 ± 0.6	**<0.001** [a]
Male sex, %	56%	36%	**0.001** [b]
Right eye, %	44%	52%	0.23 [b]
Eyes with history of previous glaucoma surgery, %	2.8%	2.0%	0.67 [b]
Mean IOP, mmHg	22.8 ± 0.7	24.3 ± 0.8	0.10 [a]
Mean number of IOP-lowering medications, n	3.1 ± 0.1	3.4 ± 0.1	0.11 [a]
Mean BCVA, LogMAR	0.25 ± 0.02	0.37 ± 0.04	0.06 [a]
Mean MD, dB	11.1 ± 1.1	11.0 ± 1.1	0.74 [a]
Mean peripapillary RNFL thickness, µm	60.6 ± 1.9	63.1 ± 1.7	0.21 [a]

POAG, primary open-angle glaucoma; PEXG, pseudoexfoliation glaucoma; IOP, intraocular pressure; BCVA, best corrected visual acuity; MD, mean defect; RNFL, retinal nerve fiber layer. p values less than 0.05 are in bold. [a] Mann–Whitney U test; [b] chi-square test.

3.1. Intraocular Pressure

At 1 day after surgery, the mean IOP decreased to 4.9 ± 0.4 mmHg in the POAG group and to 6.1 ± 0.6 mmHg in the PEXG group (Table 2; Figure 1). In the POAG cohort, mean IOP values increased until 3 months, while in the PEXG group, they increased until 1 year after DS surgery. Using the Wilcoxon signed-rank test, no significant differences in the mean IOP were found in the POAG cohort between 3 months and 5 years postoperatively ($p = 0.50$) and between 1 and 5 years postoperatively in the PEXG cohort ($p = 0.50$). Mean IOP values at 5 years reached 13.3 ± 0.6 mmHg and 16.6 ± 1.2 mmHg in the POAG and PEXG groups. Within groups, every difference in follow-up measurements compared to baseline was of statistical significance ($p < 0.001$), but no statistically significant differences between the POAG and PEXG cohorts were assessed at any of the analyzed timepoints. Five years after surgery, the mean IOP decrease was 41% ± 4% in the POAG group and 31% ± 6% in the PEXG group compared to baseline.

Table 2. Development of mean intraocular pressure and number of glaucoma medications during 5 years of follow-up after deep sclerectomy, including patients who underwent secondary glaucoma surgeries.

Timepoint	IOP, mmHg			Number of Medications, *n*		
	POAG	PEXG	p [a]	POAG	PEXG	p [a]
Preoperative	22.8 ± 0.7	24.3 ± 0.8	0.10	3.1 ± 0.1	3.4 ± 0.1	0.11
1 day	4.9 ± 0.4	6.1 ± 0.6	0.46	0.1 ± 0.04	0.1 ± 0.05	0.91
1 month	10.5 ± 0.5	11.4 ± 0.5	0.12	0.02 ± 0.02	0.04 ± 0.02	0.31
3 months	13.3 ± 0.8	13.6 ± 0.7	0.54	0.1 ± 0.1	0.1 ± 0.1	0.75
6 months	13.3 ± 0.6	13.2 ± 0.8	0.96	0.3 ± 0.1	0.5 ± 0.1	0.14
1 year	13.9 ± 1.0	16.2 ± 1.0	0.05	0.7 ± 0.2	0.8 ± 0.2	0.41
2 years	13.7 ± 0.6	15.2 ± 1.0	0.54	1.0 ± 0.2	1.1 ± 0.2	0.58
3 years	13.6 ± 0.7	16.8 ± 1.4	0.19	1.6 ± 0.3	1.4 ± 0.2	0.68
5 years	13.3 ± 0.6	16.6 ± 1.2	0.17	1.7 ± 0.3	1.7 ± 0.2	0.99

IOP, intraocular pressure; POAG, primary open-angle glaucoma; PEXG, pseudoexfoliation glaucoma. [a] Comparison between two groups was performed using Mann–Whitney U test.

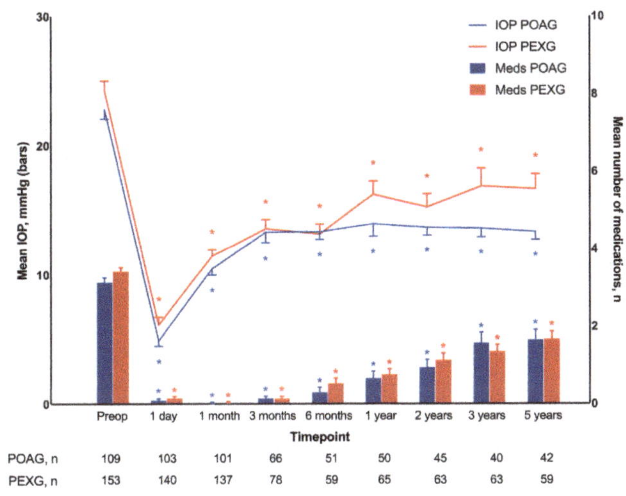

Figure 1. Development of mean intraocular pressure and number of glaucoma medications during 5 years of follow-up after deep sclerectomy in primary open-angle glaucoma and pseudoexfoliation glaucoma groups. IOP, intraocular pressure; POAG, primary open-angle glaucoma; PEXG, pseudoexfoliation glaucoma; Meds, number of glaucoma medications; Preop, preoperative. * indicates $p \leq 0.001$ (Wilcoxon signed-rank test compared to preoperative values within groups).

3.2. Number of Intraocular Pressure-Lowering Medications

At 1 day after DS, the mean number of applied IOP-lowering medications decreased to 0.1 $\pm$ 0.1 in the POAG group and to 0.1 $\pm$ 0.1 in the PEXG group (Table 2; Figure 1). Afterwards, increases in the mean number of applied IOP-lowering medications were found in both treatment groups. At 5 years after surgery, it reached 1.7 $\pm$ 0.3 and 1.7 $\pm$ 0.2 mmHg in the POAG and PEXG cohorts, respectively. Results for each follow-up visit compared to baseline values showed differences in statistical significance ($p \leq 0.001$), but no significant difference was found between cohorts for any of the analyzed timepoints. After 5 years, the mean number of IOP-lowering medications applied was reduced by 47% $\pm$ 9% in the POAG group and 51% $\pm$ 7% in the PEXG group compared to baseline before DS.

3.3. Postoperative Interventions

The number of postoperative interventions in the POAG and PEXG cohorts during 5 years of follow-up after DS is shown in Table 3. As was the case for each individual procedure, no statistically significant difference between groups was observed for the total number of interventions ($p = 0.35$). Some eyes underwent a single type of corrective procedure more than once. A total of 51% of POAG eyes underwent at least one of these procedures compared to 61% of the PEXG eyes, with no significant difference between the two cohorts (chi-square test: $p = 0.11$).

Table 3. Number of postoperative interventions during 5 years of follow-up after deep sclerectomy.

Postoperative Intervention	POAG Number of Eyes	%	PEXG Number of Eyes	%	*p*
Iridoplasties	4	4	16	7	0.55
Bleb needlings	11	9	24	11	0.75
Goniopunctures	34	28	63	37	0.24
5-FU injections	78	32	115	35	0.97
Open surgical revisions	6	6	15	10	0.21
Total	133	51	233	61	0.35

POAG, primary open-angle glaucoma; PEXG, pseudoexfoliation glaucoma; 5-FU, 5-fluorouracil. Comparison between two groups were performed using chi-square test.

3.4. Surgical Success Rates

The percentage of eyes with complete surgical success at 1 year was 54% for POAG and 39% for PEXG, with no significant difference ($p = 0.11$). At 3 years, success rates dropped to 29% for POAG and 28% for PEXG, which is still not significantly different ($p = 0.89$). By 5 years, 33% of POAG eyes and 12% of PEXG eyes achieved complete surgical success, with a significant difference ($p = 0.01$). At 1 year, 72% of POAG eyes and 55% of PEXG eyes achieved qualified surgical success, with no significant difference between the groups ($p = 0.06$). At 3 years, the success rates were 55% for POAG and 59% for PEXG, also not significantly different ($p = 0.69$). By 5 years, 63% of POAG eyes and 40% of PEXG eyes had qualified success, showing a statistically significant difference ($p = 0.03$). IOP changes comparing baseline to follow-up results measured 5 years after DS are visualized in two scatter plots in Figure 2.

3.5. Secondary Glaucoma Surgeries

In the POAG group, three cyclophotocoagulations, five TEs, one PreserFlo MicroShunt implantation, and two Baerveldt Glaucoma valve implantations were performed during the 5 years following DS. Meanwhile, nine cyclophotocoagulations, nineteen TEs, four PreserFlo MicroShunt implantations, one Baerveldt Glaucoma valve implantation, and seven XEN Gel Stent implantations were observed in the PEXG group after DS during the 5 years of follow-up. Some eyes underwent more than one of these procedures during the 5 years after DS. These cumulated to a total number of 12 secondary glaucoma surgeries in the POAG cohort and 40 in the PEXG cohort during the 5 years of follow-up, with a statistically significant difference between groups ($p = 0.04$). A total of 8% of POAG eyes underwent at least one of these procedures compared to 21% of the PEXG eyes, and a significant difference between the two cohorts was found (chi-square test: $p = 0.01$).

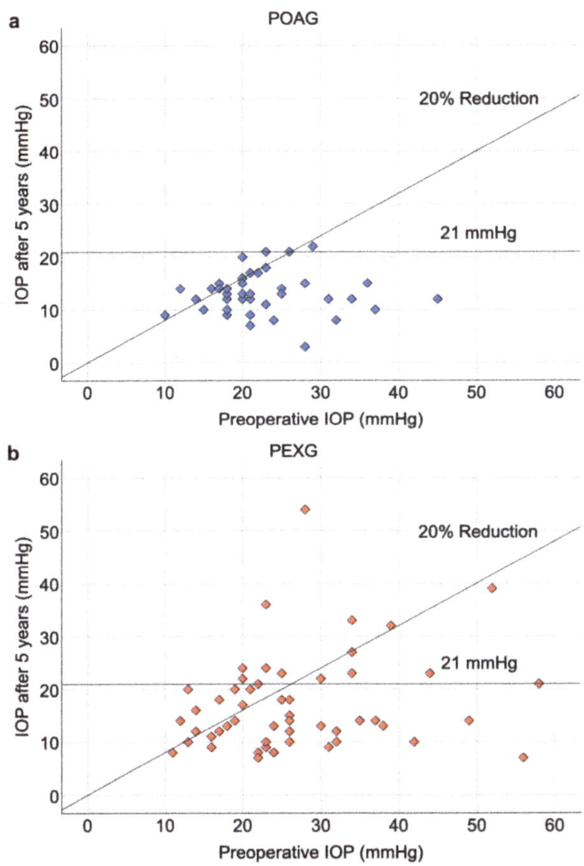

Figure 2. Scatter plots of IOP (mmHg) preoperatively and 5 years after deep sclerectomy in primary open-angle glaucoma (**a**) and pseudoexfoliation glaucoma (**b**) groups, including patients who underwent secondary glaucoma surgeries. Cases that achieved an IOP reduction equal to or greater than 20% from baseline values and cases that had a resulting IOP lower than 21 mmHg after 5 years are visualized under the respective lines. IOP, intraocular pressure; POAG, primary open-angle glaucoma; PEXG, pseudoexfoliation glaucoma.

3.6. Best Corrected Visual Acuity and Visual Field Mean Defect

The mean BCVA was 0.25 ± 0.02 logMAR and 0.37 ± 0.04 logMAR in the POAG and PEXG cohorts at baseline before surgery (Figure 3). At 1 day, the mean BCVA worsened to 0.83 ± 0.05 logMAR in the POAG group and 0.91 ± 0.05 logMAR in the PEXG group, and the inter-group difference was not of statistical significance ($p = 0.29$). Both cohorts experienced improvements afterwards, but more moderately in the PEXG group; at 3 months, BCVA reached 0.28 ± 0.04 logMAR and 0.49 ± 0.06 logMAR, respectively, with a significant difference between the two cohorts ($p = 0.02$). The BCVA worsened again in both groups later and diverged significantly at 5 years ($p = 0.04$), with the mean values reaching 0.34 ± 0.08 logMAR and 0.60 ± 0.09 logMAR in the POAG and PEXG groups.

The development of visual field mean defects is shown in Figure 4. At 5 years, MDs remained stable compared to the preoperative values at baseline in the POAG group (12.9 ± 1.6 dB, $p = 0.08$), while values significantly worsened in the PEXG group (15.0 ± 1.4 dB, $p = 0.02$). A statistically significant difference between cohorts was absent at all the analyzed post-surgical timepoints.

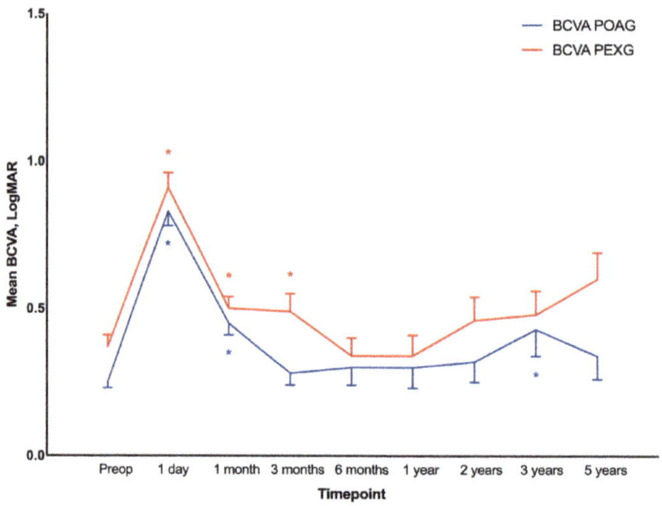

	Preop	1 day	1 month	3 months	6 months	1 year	2 years	3 years	5 years
POAG									
n	109	103	101	66	51	50	45	40	42
mean	0.25	0.83	0.45	0.28	0.30	0.30	0.32	0.43	0.34
SEM	0.02	0.05	0.04	0.04	0.06	0.07	0.07	0.09	0.08
PEXG									
n	153	140	137	78	59	65	63	63	59
mean	0.37	0.91	0.50	0.49	0.34	0.34	0.46	0.48	0.60
SEM	0.04	0.05	0.04	0.06	0.06	0.07	0.08	0.08	0.09
p	0.06	0.29	0.42	**0.02**	0.97	0.97	0.38	0.78	**0.04**

Figure 3. Development of best corrected visual acuity during 5 years of follow-up after deep sclerectomy in primary open-angle glaucoma and pseudoexfoliation glaucoma groups. BCVA, best corrected visual acuity; POAG, primary open-angle glaucoma; PEXG, pseudoexfoliation glaucoma; Preop, preoperative; SEM, standard mean error. Comparison between baseline and follow-ups within groups was performed using Wilcoxon signed-rank test (* indicates $p < 0.05$). Comparison between groups was performed using Mann–Whitney U test (p values of less than 0.05 are in bold).

3.7. Peripapillary Retinal Nerve Fiber Layer Thickness

Mean peripapillary RNFL thickness was 60.6 ± 1.9 µm in the POAG and 63.1 ± 1.7 µm in the PEXG cohort at baseline (Figure 4). At 1 year after surgery, the mean peripapillary RNFL thickness decreased significantly in both POAG ($p = 0.02$) and PEXG ($p = 0.03$) groups compared to baseline, reaching 57.3 ± 2.9 µm and 60.0 ± 2.3 µm, respectively. Afterwards, it remained stable in both cohorts, with no statistically significant difference found using the Wilcoxon signed-rank test between measured values at 1 and 2 years (POAG: $p = 0.46$, PEXG: $p = 0.68$), at 2 and 3 years (POAG: $p = 0.40$, PEXG: $p = 0.14$), and at 3 and 5 years postoperatively (POAG: $p = 0.98$, PEXG: $p = 0.13$). Overall, after 5 years, the mean peripapillary RNFL thickness had a reduction of 11% ± 5% in the POAG cohort ($p < 0.001$) and 8% ± 5% in the PEXG cohort ($p < 0.001$) compared to preoperative values. Nevertheless, a statistically significant difference between groups was absent at every timepoint. Furthermore, a correlation analysis indicated no significant association between changes in IOP and changes in peripapillary RNFL thickness after 5 years (Pearson correlation coefficient: 0.23, $p = 0.05$).

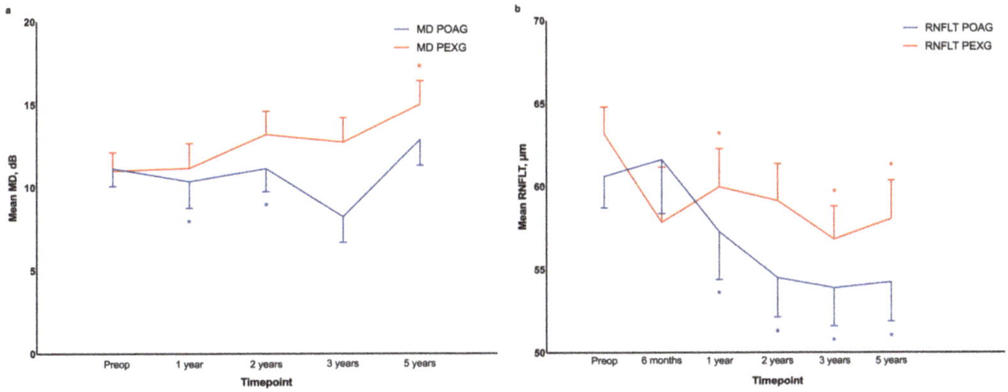

a	Preop	1 year	2 years	3 years	5 years
POAG					
n	39	20	24	13	18
mean	11.1	10.4	11.1	8.2	12.9
SEM	1.1	1.6	1.4	1.6	1.6
PEXG					
n	44	24	26	28	26
mean	11.0	11.6	13.2	12.7	15.0
SEM	1.1	1.5	1.4	1.5	1.4
p	0.74	0.61	0.26	0.07	0.32

b	Preop	6 months	1 year	2 years	3 years	5 years
POAG						
n	99	35	37	39	30	41
mean	60.6	61.6	57.3	54.5	53.9	54.2
SEM	1.9	3.2	2.9	2.7	2.3	2.4
PEXG						
n	126	23	48	51	48	49
mean	63.1	57.8	60.0	59.1	56.8	58.0
SEM	1.7	3.3	2.3	2.2	2.0	2.3
p	0.21	0.47	0.55	0.16	0.42	0.31

Figure 4. Development of visual field mean defects (**a**) and peripapillary retinal nerve fiber layer thickness (**b**) during 5 years of follow-up after deep sclerectomy in primary open-angle glaucoma and pseudoexfoliation glaucoma groups. MD, mean defect; RNFLT, retinal nerve fiber layer thickness; POAG, primary open-angle glaucoma; PEXG, pseudoexfoliation glaucoma; Preop, preoperative; SEM, standard mean error. Comparison between baseline and follow-ups within groups was performed using Wilcoxon signed-rank test (* indicates $p < 0.05$). Comparison between groups was performed using Mann–Whitney U test; p values are reported in last row.

Because of the statistically significant difference in mean age at surgery between the POAG and PEXG groups ($p < 0.001$), a correlation analysis was conducted to understand if this factor affected any difference in outcomes. The results of this analysis are shown in Table 4. The Pearson correlation coefficient was calculated for the age at surgery and each of the following differences in outcomes after 5 years: the mean IOP, the mean number of IOP-lowering medications, the total number of postoperative interventions, the total number of secondary major glaucoma surgeries, the mean BCVA, MDs, and the mean peripapillary RNFL thickness. The point biserial correlation coefficient was calculated between the age at surgery and the achievement of qualified and complete surgical success at 5 years. Only the difference in the MD after 5 years was found to be weakly [26] positively associated with patient age (0.49, $p = 0.02$). No other factor showed any significant correlation.

Table 4. Analysis of correlation between age at surgery and 5-year outcomes.

Outcome	Correlation Coefficient	p *
Δ mean IOP, mmHg	0.009 [a]	0.93
Δ mean number of IOP-lowering medications, *n*	−0.12 [a]	0.26
Δ mean BCVA, LogMAR	0.14 [a]	0.19
Δ mean MD, dB	0.49 [a]	**0.02**
Δ mean RNFL thickness, µm	−0.07 [a]	0.52
Total number of postoperative interventions, *n*	−0.06 [a]	0.38
Total number of secondary glaucoma surgeries, *n*	−0.05 [a]	0.42
Number of eyes that achieved complete success	0.009 [b]	0.93
Number of eyes that achieved qualified success	0.13 [b]	0.22

IOP, intraocular pressure; BCVA, best corrected visual acuity; MD, mean defect; RNFL, retinal nerve fiber layer. p values of less than 0.05 are in bold. [a] Pearson; [b] point biserial; * two-tailed test.

4. Discussion

Our analysis demonstrated that in the short term after surgery, DS is equally effective in decreasing IOP and the number of IOP-lowering medications in POAG and PEXG cases. This led to comparable results for complete and qualified success at 1 and 3 years after surgery while stabilizing BCVA and visual field MD in both groups. However, in the medium term, the percentage of PEXG cases meeting success criteria decreased strongly and the difference to the POAG group became statistically significant at 5 years after surgery. Also, the number of eyes needing secondary glaucoma surgery was larger in the PEXG group compared to the POAG group ($p = 0.01$). Additionally, RNFL decrease continued until 1 year after DS in both groups, stabilizing thereafter in both POAG and PEXG eyes.

These results are similar to previous findings by Ollikainen et al. [17], suggesting no significant difference in IOP values between 31 POAG and 37 PEXG eyes 3 years after DS. Another study by Studeny et al. [18] found a significant IOP reduction in 10 PEXG patients 2 years after DS performed with a T-flux implant, with mean values decreasing from 36.8 ± 8.7 mmHg to 14.8 ± 2.4 mmHg (median values, ±standard deviation (SD), $p < 0.001$). The change in IOP was larger than our observed reduction at the same timepoint, which accounted for a decrease from 24.3 ± 0.8 mmHg to 15.2 ± 1.0 mmHg ($p < 0.001$). In both cohorts, the postoperative phase of scarring activity induced a delayed increase in IOP after an initial period of rapid IOP reduction [27]. The strong IOP reduction in the early postoperative period may be due to the surgical strategy used in our clinic. During surgery, strong filtration is allowed from the beginning, aiming at borderline hypotensive IOP levels at the end of the procedure. Usually, only a few scleral flap sutures are used with very low tension to minimize interference with aqueous humor flow. Excessive hypotension is not common and manageable if present. Nevertheless, laser suture lysis and 5-FU injections are a common part of the postoperative regimen in our clinic.

Our results concerning the necessity for the application of IOP-lowering medications after surgery were similar to a previous study by Ollikainen et al. [19], which also found no difference regarding the reduction in the number of glaucoma medications between 31 POAG and 37 PEXG eyes up to 1 year after DS. The change in the PEXG group at 5 years after DS (medication reduction from 3.4 ± 0.1 to 1.7 ± 0.2, $p < 0.001$) was more moderate compared to a study by Mendrinos et al. [20], where 22 PEXG eyes had a reduction from 2.4 ± 0.67 to 0.59 ± 0.85 after a follow-up of 48.5 ± 12.2 months (mean values, ±SD, $p < 0.0001$).

The percentage of eyes undergoing postoperative interventions was comparable in both groups. This was similar to a previous study by Drolsum [21] that reported a non-significant difference in cases which underwent goniopuncture in 27 POAG (30%; mean follow-up of 43 months) and 28 PEXG eyes (32%; mean follow-up of 45 months). In comparison, our observed percentage of cases with goniopunctures was 28% and 37% in the POAG and PEXG cohorts, respectively, which also lacked a difference in statistical significance between both groups (chi-square test: $p = 0.10$).

However, our observations regarding differences in re-operation rates showed that 8% of POAG eyes and 21% of PEXG eyes ($p = 0.01$) underwent secondary major glaucoma surgery during the 5 years of follow-up after DS, which suggests an overall worse postoperative course in the PEXG cohort. In comparison, Rekonen et al. [22] reported a 10% rate in POAG eyes and 18% rate in PEXG eyes during a follow-up of 18 months after DS (no statistically significant difference between groups). Interestingly, at 18 months after DS, the different rate of necessary major secondary glaucoma surgery between our POAG and PEXG cohorts was also not of statistical significance (4% POAG; 6% PEXG; chi-square test: $p = 0.42$). Only analysis of longer follow-up results in our study showed diverging re-operation rates between POAG and PEXG cohorts with differences in statistical significance. Drolsum [21] and Mendrinos et al. [20], who analyzed longer postoperative follow-up periods, did not report detailed information concerning re-operation rates.

The analysis regarding the progression of visual field defects was affected by the statistically significant older mean age at surgery of the PEXG cohort. Studies by Konstas et al. [28] and Nakano et al. [29] have reported that PEXG patients tend to be older than POAG patients, indicating that this age difference may be an epidemiological difference rather than an inclusion bias. Age did not influence other outcomes. Although the correlation between this factor and the changes in SAP results after 5 years was weak, it may have nonetheless played a role in shaping the observed findings, contributing to the assessed worsened visual field defects among PEXG patients 5 years after DS compared to preoperative values. Nevertheless, after 5 years, no statistically significant difference was found between groups for this outcome, which is relevant in the overall analysis, as a less compromised visual field is directly correlated with a higher quality of life [30]. A comparable reduction in peripapillary RNFL thickness was recorded for both cohorts, which stabilized approximately after the first postoperative year and was not associated with the resulting IOP changes after surgery. The absence of this correlation has already been described in the literature [31]. In a prospective trial by Rebolleda et al. [32], visual field global indices and peripapillary RNFL thickness were found to be comparable to preoperative values 6 months after DS in 34 patients with unspecified glaucoma. Our initial observations for these outcomes in PEXG eyes were similar, with no significant postoperative changes at 6 months in peripapillary RNFL thickness ($p = 0.19$) but with later worsening courses for peripapillary RNFL thickness ($p < 0.001$) and for the mean defect values of SAP ($p = 0.02$) after 5 years.

Similarly, the performed analysis showed worse outcomes for success levels among PEXG patients 5 years after DS, as POAG patients tended to achieve higher rates for both qualified and complete success. These outcomes may underestimate existing results due to the large rate of dropouts during follow-up. This assumes that patients with more favorable outcomes may be less likely to attend control examinations, as has already been described for other ophthalmic procedures before, such as strabismus surgery [33]. It also assumes that patients who experience worse subjective symptoms may indeed have less favorable objective outcomes, as Viswanathan et al. have observed for visual field deterioration in particular [34], and might therefore worsen observed results if they are more likely to attend follow-up. The aforementioned study by Studeny et al. [18] indicated complete and qualified success rates of 85% and 100%, respectively, in 20 PEXG eyes 1 year after DS, which were noticeably higher than ours at the same timepoint (39% for complete success and 55% for qualified success). Furthermore, Ollikainen et al. [17] reported no significant difference for both complete and qualified success rates between 31 POAG eyes (74% and 74%, respectively) and 37 PEXG eyes (73% and 73%) 3 years after surgery. These values are higher than our findings at the same timepoint but are in line with our results concerning a comparison between both groups, as we also could not find differences in statistical significance between groups 3 years after DS. A longer trial by Drolsum [21] showed the absence of statistically significant differences concerning the achievement of complete success after a mean follow-up time of approximately 4 years, with 50.0% in PEXG eyes compared to 33.3% in POAG eyes respecting the criteria.

The inferior success rates, together with worse BCVA, ultimately led to overall worse results of DS in the PEXG cohort compared to the POAG cohort at 5 years after surgery, even though other clinical outcomes were indeed similar between both groups. Other studies indicated before that DS may be safe and useful for PEXG eyes in the medium term [17–22]. The herein presented results lightly hint towards DS being more beneficial in POAG eyes compared to PEXG over a longer follow-up period. Other surgical options for PEXG patients include TE. However, there are also conflicting results regarding the efficacy of TE in PEXG eyes [35–37], suggesting that PEXG may be more difficult to treat than POAG, regardless of therapeutic approach.

Our herein presented analysis provides detailed information about the development of anatomical (peripapillary RNFL thickness) and functional parameters (SAP indices) after DS, as well as a large quantity of other clinical data that are frequently reported in similar but mostly smaller cohorts. Moreover, we followed patients over a longer period of time, which is essential given the chronic nature of glaucoma. We also analyzed a sizeable number of patients with data originating from only one eye per participant included in the analysis, which was useful to provide statistically significant and higher quality information. Weaknesses of the study include the lack of analysis of postoperative complications, the retrospective, non-randomized, unblinded, and unicentric design, the number of patients lost to follow-up, and the multiple number of surgeons performing surgery. DS is a procedure that has been frequently performed by many surgeons at the Bern University Hospital over the years. This may lead to variations in the procedure performed. However, we did not find a high variability of postoperative outcomes in terms of IOP, medications, and success rate. Performing the herein described analyses in a larger cohort coming from multiple centers in a prospective manner could be a goal of future studies.

5. Conclusions

DS has been proven to provide comparable outcomes in PEXG and POAG eyes regarding IOP, the number of IOP-lowering medications, visual field defects, and peripapillary RNFL thickness 5 years after surgery. However, PEXG eyes were significantly more likely to require subsequent major surgical glaucoma interventions, and the complete and qualified success rates were lower after 5 years of follow-up compared to POAG eyes. Based on the results of our study, it can be argued that the long-term success of DS in eyes suffering from PEXG is lower than in those suffering from POAG. In our case, this will influence our strategy when planning surgical interventions for the treatment of glaucoma (POAG and PEXG) in the future. The presented results may help surgeons and patients make more informed choices about their treatment options. Nevertheless, more studies with larger patient cohorts are needed to evaluate this procedure and other treatment options to provide better targeted surgical care for PEXG patients.

Author Contributions: Conceptualization, J.D.U. and M.S.Z.; methodology, J.D.U.; software, X.S. and C.F.; validation, J.D.U. and X.S.; formal analysis, J.D.U. and C.F.; investigation, C.F.; resources, J.D.U. and M.S.Z.; data curation, J.D.U., C.F. and X.S.; writing—original draft preparation, C.F.; writing—review and editing, J.D.U., X.S., J.-B.L., N.U.H. and M.S.Z.; visualization, J.D.U., C.F. and X.S.; supervision, J.D.U. and M.S.Z.; project administration, J.D.U. and M.S.Z.; funding acquisition, J.D.U. and M.S.Z. All authors have read and agreed to the published version of the manuscript.

Funding: This research received no external funding.

Institutional Review Board Statement: The study was conducted in accordance with the Declaration of Helsinki and approved by the Ethics Committee of the Canton of Bern (BASEC-ID: 2022-01046; date of approval: 15 March 2023).

Informed Consent Statement: Informed consent for participants was waived due to the retrospective nature of this study.

Data Availability Statement: The datasets used for this study are available from the corresponding author upon reasonable request.

Acknowledgments: We acknowledge the support provided by the Department of Ophthalmology, Inselspital, Bern University Hospital.

Conflicts of Interest: None of the authors has any competing interests to disclose. M.S.Z.: Allergan, Bayer, Novartis, Heidelberg Engineering, Boehringer Ingelheim (all consulting and speaker's honoraria, not related to the here presented work; the funders had no role in the design of the study, in the collection, analyses, or interpretation of data, in the writing of the manuscript, or in the decision to publish the results).

References

1. Höhn, R.; Pfeiffer, N. Klassifikation, Genetik und Epidemiologie der Glaukome. *Klin. Monbl. Augenheilkd.* **2017**, *234*, 931–948. [CrossRef] [PubMed]
2. Weinreb, R.N.; Aung, T.; Medeiros, F.A. The pathophysiology and treatment of glaucoma: A review. *JAMA* **2014**, *311*, 1901–1911. [CrossRef] [PubMed]
3. Gedde, S.J.; Lind, J.T.; Wright, M.M. American Academy of Ophthalmology Preferred Practice Pattern glaucoma panel. Primary open-angle glaucoma Preferred Practice Pattern®. *Ophthalmology* **2021**, *128*, 71–150. [CrossRef] [PubMed]
4. Tham, Y.C.; Li, X.; Wong, T.Y.; Quigley, H.A.; Aung, T.; Cheng, C.Y. Global prevalence of glaucoma and projections of glaucoma burden through 2040: A systematic review and meta-analysis. *Ophthalmology* **2014**, *121*, 2081–2090. [CrossRef] [PubMed]
5. Elhawy, E.; Kamthan, G.; Dong, C.Q.; Danias, J. Pseudoexfoliation syndrome, a systemic disorder with ocular manifestations. *Hum. Genom.* **2012**, *6*, 22. [CrossRef]
6. Hicks, P.M.; Siedlecki, A.; Haaland, B.; Owen, L.A.; Au, E.; Feehan, M.; Murtaugh, M.A.; Sieminski, S.; Reynolds, A.; Lillvis, J. A global genetic epidemiological review of pseudoexfoliation syndrome. *Explor. Med.* **2021**, *2*, 527–543. [CrossRef]
7. Ritch, R.; Schlötzer-Schrehardt, U.; Konstas, A.G. Why is glaucoma associated with exfoliation syndrome? *Prog. Retin. Eye Res.* **2003**, *22*, 253–275. [CrossRef]
8. Lee, D.A.; Higginbotham, E.J. Glaucoma and its treatment: A review. *Am. J. Health-Syst. Pharm.* **2005**, *62*, 691–699. [CrossRef]
9. Rao, A.; Cruz, R.D. Trabeculectomy: Does it have a future? *Cureus* **2022**, *14*, 27834. [CrossRef]
10. Razeghinejad, M.R.; Fudemberg, S.J.; Spaeth, G.L. The changing conceptual basis of trabeculectomy: A review of past and current surgical techniques. *Surv. Ophthalmol.* **2012**, *57*, 1–25. [CrossRef]
11. Rulli, E.; Biagioli, E.; Riva, I.; Gambirasio, G.; De Simone, I.; Floriani, I.; Quaranta, L. Efficacy and safety of trabeculectomy vs nonpenetrating surgical procedures: A systematic review and meta-analysis. *JAMA Ophthalmol.* **2013**, *131*, 1573–1582. [CrossRef] [PubMed]
12. Richardson-May, J.; Alnuaimi, R.; Elbably, A.; Walker, L.; Thulasidharan, S.; Dacombe, R.; Jacob, A. Our experience of deep sclerectomy at a tertiary center in the United Kingdom over 14 years. *Cureus* **2023**, *15*, 43366. [CrossRef]
13. Klemm, M. Tiefe Sklerektomie. Eine Alternative zur Trabekulektomie. *Ophthalmologe* **2015**, *112*, 313–318. [CrossRef] [PubMed]
14. Heijl, A.; Bengtsson, B.; Hyman, L.; Leske, M.C.; Early Manifest Glaucoma Trial Group. Natural history of open-angle glaucoma. *Ophthalmology* **2009**, *116*, 2271–2276. [CrossRef] [PubMed]
15. Gottanka, J.; Flügel-Koch, C.; Martus, P.; Johnson, D.H.; Lütjen-Drecoll, E. Correlation of pseudoexfoliative material and optic nerve damage in pseudoexfoliation syndrome. *Investig. Ophthalmol. Vis. Sci.* **1997**, *38*, 2435–2446.
16. Suominen, S.M.; Harju, M.P.; Vesti, E.T. Deep sclerectomy in primary open-angle glaucoma and exfoliative glaucoma. *Eur. J. Ophthalmol.* **2016**, *26*, 568–574. [CrossRef]
17. Ollikainen, M.L.; Puustjärvi, T.J.; Rekonen, P.K.; Uusitalo, H.M.; Teräsvirta, M.E. Mitomycin C-augmented deep sclerectomy in primary open-angle glaucoma and exfoliation glaucoma: A three-year prospective study. *Acta Ophthalmol.* **2011**, *89*, 548–555. [CrossRef]
18. Studeny, P.; Baxant, A.D.; Vranova, J.; Kuchynka, P.; Pokorna, J. Deep sclerectomy with nonabsorbable implant (T-Flux) in patients with pseudoexfoliation glaucoma. *J. Ophthalmol.* **2017**, *2017*, 6923208. [CrossRef]
19. Ollikainen, M.; Puustjärvi, T.; Rekonen, P.; Uusitalo, H.; Teräsvirta, M. Mitomycin-C-augmented deep sclerectomy in patients with primary open-angle glaucoma and exfoliation glaucoma: A 1-year prospective study. *Acta Ophthalmol.* **2010**, *88*, 20–26. [CrossRef]
20. Mendrinos, E.; Mansouri, K.; Mermoud, A.; Shaarawy, T. Long-term results of deep sclerectomy with collagen implant in exfoliative glaucoma. *J. Glaucoma* **2009**, *18*, 361–367. [CrossRef]
21. Drolsum, L. Longterm follow-up after deep sclerectomy in patients with pseudoexfoliative glaucoma. *Acta Ophthalmol. Scand.* **2006**, *84*, 502–506. [CrossRef] [PubMed]
22. Rekonen, P.; Kannisto, T.; Puustjärvi, T.; Teräsvirta, M.; Uusitalo, H. Deep sclerectomy for the treatment of exfoliation and primary open-angle glaucoma. *Acta Ophthalmol. Scand.* **2006**, *84*, 507–511. [CrossRef] [PubMed]
23. Hoffer, K.J.; Aramberri, J.; Haigis, W.; Olsen, T.; Savini, G.; Shammas, H.J.; Bentow, S. Protocols for studies of intraocular lens formula accuracy. *Am. J. Ophthalmol.* **2015**, *160*, 403–405. [CrossRef] [PubMed]
24. Anand, N.; Kumar, A.; Gupta, A. Primary phakic deep sclerectomy augmented with mitomycin C: Long-term outcomes. *J. Glaucoma* **2011**, *20*, 21–27. [CrossRef]
25. Mermoud, A.; Schnyder, C.C. Nonpenetrating filtering surgery in glaucoma. *Curr. Opin. Ophthalmol.* **2000**, *11*, 151–157. [CrossRef]
26. Miot, H.A. Correlation analysis in clinical and experimental studies. *J. Vasc. Bras.* **2018**, *17*, 275–279. [CrossRef]
27. Delarive, T.; Rossier, A.; Rossier, S.; Ravinet, E.; Shaarawy, T.; Mermoud, A. Aqueous dynamic and histological findings after deep sclerectomy with collagen implant in an animal model. *Br. J. Ophthalmol.* **2003**, *87*, 1340–1344. [CrossRef]
28. Konstas, A.G.; Tsatsos, I.; Kardasopoulos, A.; Bufidis, T.; Maskaleris, G. Preoperative features of patients with exfoliation glaucoma and primary open-angle glaucoma. The AHEPA study. *Acta Ophthalmol. Scand.* **1998**, *76*, 208–212. [CrossRef]
29. Nakano, H.; Togano, T.; Sakaue, Y.; Suetaka, A.; Iikawa, R.; Nakano, R.; Fukuchi, T. Clinical features of patients with exfoliation glaucoma requiring surgical intervention. *J. Ophthalmol.* **2020**, *2020*, 9423756. [CrossRef]
30. Rossi, G.C.M.; Milano, G.; De Silvestri, A.; Savini, L.; Bosi, C.; Gambini, G.; Rama, P. Correlation between visual field index and quality of life in glaucoma patients: A new tool to screen quality of life perception? *Front. Med.* **2023**, *10*, 1214007. [CrossRef]

31. Koenig, S.F.; Hirneiss, C.W. Changes of neuroretinal rim and retinal nerve fiber layer thickness assessed by optical coherence tomography after filtration surgery in glaucomatous eyes. *Clin. Ophthalmol.* **2021**, *15*, 2335–2344. [CrossRef] [PubMed]
32. Rebolleda, G.; Muñoz-Negrete, F.J.; Noval, S. Evaluation of changes in peripapillary nerve fiber layer thickness after deep sclerectomy with optical coherence tomography. *Ophthalmology* **2007**, *114*, 488–493. [CrossRef] [PubMed]
33. Daly, C.M.; Dembinski, R.L.; Kraus, C.L. Factors leading to loss to follow-up after strabismus surgery in children. *J. AAPOS* **2021**, *25*, 142.e1–142.e4. [CrossRef]
34. Viswanathan, A.C.; McNaught, A.I.; Poinoosawmy, D.; Fontana, L.; Crabb, D.P.; Fitzke, F.W.; Hitchings, R.A. Severity and stability of glaucoma: Patient perception compared with objective measurement. *Arch. Ophthalmol.* **1999**, *117*, 450–454. [CrossRef] [PubMed]
35. Jerndal, T.; Kriisa, V. Results of trabeculectomy for pseudo-exfoliative glaucoma. A study of 52 cases. *Br. J. Ophthalmol.* **1974**, *58*, 927–930. [CrossRef] [PubMed]
36. Li, F.; Tang, G.; Zhang, H.; Yan, X.; Ma, L.; Geng, Y. The effects of trabeculectomy on pseudoexfoliation glaucoma and primary open-angle glaucoma. *J. Ophthalmol.* **2020**, *2020*, 1723691. [CrossRef]
37. Popovic, V.; Sjöstrand, J. Course of exfoliation and simplex glaucoma after primary trabeculectomy. *Br. J. Ophthalmol.* **1999**, *83*, 305–310. [CrossRef]

Journal of
Clinical Medicine

MDPI

Article

Asymmetric Glaucoma and Corresponding Hearing Impairment

Laura Antonia Meliante [1,*], Giulia Coco [1], Beatrice Francavilla [2], Matilde Bianchi [1], Gianluca Velletrani [2], Stefano Di Girolamo [2] and Gianluca Manni [1,3,*]

1 Department of Clinical Sciences and Translational Medicine, University of Rome Tor Vergata, 00133 Rome, Italy
2 Department of Otorhinolaryngology, University of Rome "Tor Vergata", 00133 Rome, Italy
3 IRCCS—Fondazione Bietti, 00184 Rome, Italy
* Correspondence: lauraantonia.meliante@ptvonline.it (L.A.M.); gianlucamanni53@gmail.com (G.M.); Tel.: +39-3484772028 (L.A.M.); +39-0620902969 (G.M.)

Abstract: Background/Objectives: This study aims to explore the potential relationship between unilateral or asymmetric glaucoma and ipsilateral hearing impairment. **Methods**: In this retrospective study, visual and hearing functions were assessed in patients with unilateral or asymmetric glaucoma. Correlations between retinal nerve fiber layer (RNFL) thickness, visual field mean deviation (MD) values, and pure tone audiometry (PTA) measurements across various frequencies were analyzed to explore potential associations between visual and ipsilateral hearing functions. Differences in PTA values between ears ipsilateral to the more affected glaucomatous eyes and the contralateral ears were studied for statistical significance. **Results**: Twenty-six patients with unilateral or asymmetric glaucoma were included in the study. Significant differences in hearing thresholds between the ears corresponding to the more severely glaucomatous eyes and the contralateral ears were found at 0.7, 1, 1.5, and 3 kHz ($p < 0.05$). Additionally, a statistically significant difference was observed in the speech frequencies (0.5, 0.7, 1, 1.5, 2, 3, and 4 kHz) between ears corresponding to glaucomatous or more affected glaucomatous eyes and the contralateral ears ($p = 0.016$). Furthermore, a moderately positive correlation was found between differences in MD and PTA values at 0.125 kHz ($r = 0.50$; $p = 0.01$). **Conclusions**: This study highlights a potential association between unilateral or asymmetric glaucoma and ipsilateral hearing impairment, particularly at speech-relevant frequencies. These findings underscore the importance of integrated sensory assessment in the management of glaucoma patients, suggesting that early detection and intervention for concurrent hearing loss could enhance overall quality of life.

Keywords: glaucoma; unilateral glaucoma; asymmetric glaucoma; hearing loss; hearing impairment

1. Introduction

Glaucoma, a leading cause of irreversible blindness worldwide, primarily affects the optic nerve, leading to progressive vision loss [1]. A few studies and reviews have examined the potential association of glaucoma and hearing impairment [2]. This relationship could be explained by several potential mechanisms. Glaucoma and hearing loss share common pathogenic factors, including vascular impairment and neurodegeneration [2]. Glaucoma is characterized by the degeneration of the optic nerve, the thinning of retinal nerve fibers, and the loss of retinal ganglion cells, frequently associated with vascular abnormalities such as diminished perfusion pressure and impaired vascular autoregulation [3–7]. Similarly, sensorineural hearing loss (SNHL) results from cochlear and auditory nerve damage, influenced by microvascular alterations causing ischemic injury to inner ear structures [8,9].

Understanding the broader implications of glaucoma is crucial for developing comprehensive management strategies that address all aspects of patients' quality of life (QoL). Although most affected patients do not report any specific symptoms or vision loss initially, glaucoma can adversely affect patients' QoL and ability to perform visually related activities, even when they are unaware of their diagnosis [10].

Hearing loss (HL), like vision loss, is a major public health concern that significantly affects daily functioning and social interactions. Effective communication relies heavily on auditory perception, and any impairment can lead to social isolation, depression, and diminished overall well-being [10]. Unlike vision impairment, which primarily affects spatial navigation and interaction with the physical environment, hearing loss hinders social engagement and the ability to participate in conversations [10]. When both vision and hearing impairments co-occur, the negative impact on physical and mental health is compounded, leading to a greater overall decline in QoL than when either impairment occurs alone [10].

Previous studies have identified associations between glaucoma and various forms of HL, particularly in conditions such as pseudoexfoliation syndrome. However, the relationship between primary open-angle glaucoma, pigmentary glaucoma, and auditory deficits has received limited attention [2]. The potential association between unilateral glaucoma and ipsilateral HL remains underexplored. Additionally, the correlations between retinal nerve fiber layer (RNFL) thickness and pure tone audiometry (PTA) values have not been thoroughly investigated. Exploring these relationships is essential for understanding whether the ear ipsilateral to the glaucomatous eye or the one affected by more severe glaucoma exhibits poorer hearing, and for elucidating the potential connections between ophthalmic and auditory health.

This study aims to fill these gaps by evaluating the potential relationship between unilateral or asymmetric glaucoma and hearing impairment ipsilateral to the more affected eye. Additionally, we aimed to investigate whether the presence of glaucoma more noticeably affects auditory performance at speech-relevant frequencies, potentially further impacting patients' QoL.

2. Materials and Methods

In this retrospective study, visual and hearing functions were assessed in patients followed in the Glaucoma Unit at Policlinico Tor Vergata in Rome.

2.1. Inclusion and Exclusion Criteria

Patients were included if they had either a diagnosis of unilateral glaucoma or a strongly asymmetric glaucoma. Unilateral glaucoma was defined by the presence in only one eye of (i) glaucomatous defects in the Humphrey 24-2, 30-2, or 10-2 computerized visual field (VF), defined as three or more contiguous points with $p < 0.05$ or two or more contiguous points with $p < 0.01$, or a difference of 10 dB across the nasal horizontal midline in two or more adjacent points, or mean deviation (MD) worse than −5 dB; (ii) ophthalmoscopic diagnosis of glaucoma based on the detection of a glaucomatous optic disc at the fundus examination performed by a glaucoma specialist; (iii) positive Hood glaucoma report at the optical coherence tomography (OCT) for glaucoma. When both eyes met the diagnostic criteria for glaucoma, strongly asymmetric glaucoma was defined in case of: (i) MD difference $\geq$ 3 dB between the two eyes; (ii) cup-to-disc ratio (C/D) difference $\geq$ 0.2 between the two eyes; and (iii) peripapillary retinal nerve fiber layer-global (RNFL-g) thickness difference $\geq$ 20 μm between the two eyes, measured on OCT.

Additional inclusion criteria were the availability of data regarding VF examination, fundus examination, Hood glaucoma report, and PTA at 0.125, 0.250, 0.500, 0.700, 1, 1.5, 2, 3, 4, 6, and 8 kHz, all performed within one year.

Exclusion criteria were applied for both ophthalmological and ear, nose, and throat (ENT) reasons. Ophthalmological exclusion criteria included the presence of unilateral glaucoma secondary to trauma, surgical procedures, ocular inflammation, and/or infections, and patients with angle-closure glaucoma. ENT exclusion criteria included a history of ear or vestibular disorders, any previous ear surgeries, prolonged occupational exposure to high noise levels, a history of ear trauma or chronic ear infections, and the use of medications known to have ototoxic effects.

2.2. Ocular Examination and Glaucoma Diagnosis

All participants underwent full ophthalmological examination by a glaucoma specialist, including best corrected visual acuity (BCVA), Goldman applanation tonometry measurements, as well as anterior slit-lamp biomicroscopy and fundus examination. Visual field assessments were conducted using a Humphrey Field Analyzer HFAII-740i and HFAIII (Carl Zeiss Meditec, Inc., Dublin, CA, USA), employing a 24-2 threshold program with the Swedish Interactive Threshold Algorithm (SITA) standard testing strategy. Optical coherence tomography (OCT) was performed using the Spectralis OCT (Heidelberg Engineering, Heidelberg, Germany) and the Hood glaucoma report was generated.

2.3. Otolaryngologic Examination and Audiometric Assessment

Hearing thresholds for both ears were assessed using the pure-tone audiometry (PTA) at the following frequencies: 0.125, 0.250, 0.500, 0.700, 1, 1.5, 2, 3, 4, 6, and 8 kHz. A comprehensive otological evaluation and otoscopy were conducted by an experienced otolaryngologist.

2.4. Statistical Analysis

The Shapiro–Wilk test was used to determine the normality of PTA, mean deviation (MD), and RNFL values. Depending on the data distribution, either Pearson's or Spearman's correlation coefficients were used to assess the relationship between PTA values at the tested frequencies and RNFL values and PTA and MD values. Correlations of inter-eye differences in MD and RNFL and inter-ear differences in PTA were also analyzed to further explore potential associations. Paired *t*-tests and Wilcoxon's matched-pair signed-rank tests were used to compare PTA values between ears ipsilateral to the glaucomatous eye, or the most damaged one in asymmetrical cases, and the contralateral ears. All statistical analyses were performed with the software R (version 4.4.0 GUI 1.80 Big Sur ARM build released on 24 April 2024) and a two-sided *p*-value of 0.05 was considered for statistical significance.

The study followed the tenets of the Declaration of Helsinki and was approved by the local ethical committee.

3. Results

Twenty-six patients were included in the study. Twenty-three had primary open-angle glaucoma (POAG), two had pigmentary glaucoma, and one had pseudoexfoliative glaucoma (PXG). The mean age was 71.69 ± 9.54 and 18 of the patients were male (69.2%).

All patients had unilateral (n = 21) or asymmetric glaucoma (n = 5), affecting the right eye in 11 cases and the left eye in 15 cases. All 26 patients included in this study were Italian and of Caucasian ethnicity.

3.1. Ophthalmological Characteristics

The glaucomatous or more severely glaucomatous eyes and the contralateral eyes showed significant differences in several key parameters, as outlined in Table 1. The mean number of hypotensive drops administered was 1.19 ± 1.06 for the glaucomatous or more severely affected eye and 1.35 ± 1.06 for the less glaucomatous eye. Additionally, the mean number of active pharmaceutical ingredients used was 1.42 ± 1.30 for the more glaucomatous eyes, compared to 1.69 ± 1.43 for the contralateral eyes. In terms of surgical interventions, 12 out of 26 eyes in the more glaucomatous group had undergone trabeculectomy or trabeculectomy combined with phacoemulsification. Among these, 2 patients required revision surgery following trabeculectomy, and 1 patient underwent re-trabeculectomy. In contrast, none of the eyes in the non-glaucomatous or less affected glaucomatous group had undergone any surgical interventions for glaucoma.

Table 1. Mean values of baseline ophthalmological parameters in glaucomatous or more severely glaucomatous eyes and the contralateral eyes.

	More Severely/ Glaucomatous Eyes	Less Severely/ Non-Glaucomatous Eyes	*p*-Value
RNFL (micron)	55.88 ± 12.87	93.66 ± 8.93	0.00 [P]
BCVA (logMAR)	0.17 ± 0.19	0.08 ± 0.18	0.02 [W]
MD (dB)	−12.8 ± 10.58	−0.38 ± 1.83	0.06 [P]
IOP (mmHg)	14 ± 6.3	14 ± 3.1	0.45 [W]

BCVA: best corrected visual acuity; MD: mean deviation; IOP: intraocular pressure; [P]: paired *t*-test; RNFL: retinal nerve fiber layer thickness; [W]: Wilcoxon's signed-rank test.

3.2. Pure Tone Audiometry (PTA)

The average PTA values, expressed in dB across various frequencies, are illustrated in Figure 1.

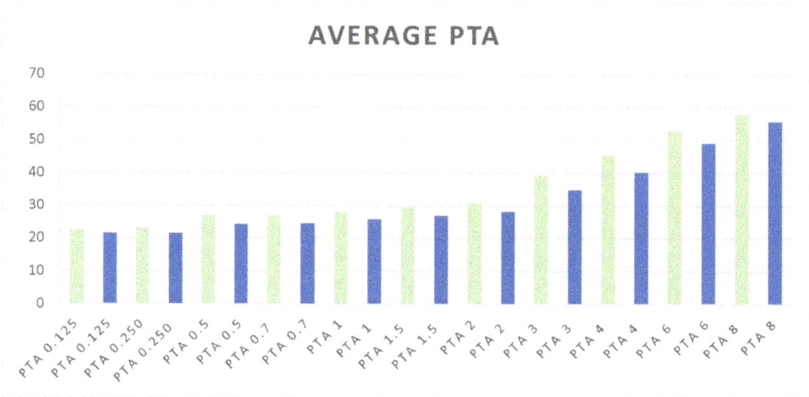

Figure 1. Average of PTA values at different frequencies. Green bars represent PTA values (kHz) for ears corresponding to glaucomatous or more affected glaucomatous eyes, while blue bars represent PTA values for ears corresponding to non-glaucomatous or less affected glaucomatous eyes. The PTA frequencies range from 0.125 kHz to 8 kHz.

These values compare the ears corresponding to glaucomatous or more affected glaucomatous eyes with the contralateral ears, providing a visual representation of hearing thresholds.

3.3. Paired t-Tests and Wilcoxon's Signed-Rank Tests

A Wilcoxon signed-rank test was performed for non-normally distributed data (PTA 0.125, 0.250, 0.7, 1, 2, 3, 6, 8 kHz). Although no statistically significant differences were found at 0.125 kHz or 0.250 kHz (mean differences of 0.96 dB and 1.73 dB, respectively, with small effect sizes of 0.10 and 0.17), statistically significant differences were found at 0.7 kHz (p = 0.02), 1 kHz (p = 0.03), and 3 kHz (p = 0.02); at these frequencies, the mean differences were 2.88 dB, 2.31 dB, and 4.42 dB, respectively, with confidence intervals indicating moderate effect sizes (Cohen's d = 0.22, 0.18, and 0.20) suggesting that patients with unilateral or asymmetric glaucoma may have hypoacusis in the corresponding ear at these frequencies, thus identifying a potential specific frequency range where glaucoma may impact auditory function. A paired t-test was performed for normally distributed data (PTA 0.5, 1.5, 4 kHz). The result of the paired t-test at the frequency of 1.5 kHz shows a p-value of 0.04, which is statistically significant, with a mean difference of 2.69 dB (95% CI [0.18, 5.20]) and a small effect size (Cohen's d = 0.18), indicating that hearing thresholds are likely to be affected by glaucoma at this frequency. This result further supports the hypothesis that there may be specific frequencies where glaucoma affects hearing thresholds more noticeably. At higher frequencies, such as 2 kHz and 4 kHz, while there were notable mean differences of 2.69 dB and 5.19 dB, the clinical relevance is less clear due to wider confidence intervals and smaller effect sizes, particularly at 4 kHz (Cohen's d = 0.23). Similarly, at 6 kHz and 8 kHz, neither the statistical tests nor the effect sizes (Cohen's d = 0.14 and 0.07, respectively) suggest any significant difference in auditory function between glaucomatous and non-glaucomatous ears. The results of the paired *t*-tests and Wilcoxon's signed-rank tests, summarized in Table 2, provide detailed insights into the differences in hearing thresholds between glaucomatous and non-glaucomatous ears across various frequencies. The table includes the mean PTA values (±SD) for both groups at each tested frequency, along with the mean differences of PTA between the two groups, 95% confidence intervals, and Cohen's d as a measure of effect size.

Table 2. Paired *t*-test and Wilcoxon's signed-rank test results.

PTA Frequency [kHz]	PTA G (Mean ± SD) [dB]	PTA NG (Mean ± SD) [dB]	Mean Difference (PTA G-PTA NG) ± SD [dB]	95% CI	Effect Size (Cohen's d)	*p*-Value
0.125 [W]	22.5 ± 9.08	21.54 ± 9.77	0.96 ± 8.25	[−2.37; 4.29]	0.10	0.56
0.250 [W]	23.27 ± 9.79	21.54 ± 10.93	1.73 ± 7.47	[−1.28; 4.75]	10.37	0.24
0.5 [P]	27.1 ± 11.85	24.23 ± 11.02	2.88 ± 7.50	[−1.47; 5.91]	11.44	0.06
0.7 [W]	27.71 ± 13.75	24.58 ± 12.24	2.88 ± 6.02	[0.44; 5.31]	13.03	0.02 *
1 [W]	28.08 ± 12.66	25.77 ± 13.09	2.31 ± 6.14	[0.23; 4.38]	12.88	0.03 *
1.5 [P]	29.79 ± 15.29	26.88 ± 14.36	2.69 ± 6.20	[0.18; 5.20]	14.83	0.04 *
2 [W]	30.96 ± 16.79	28.27 ± 15.29	2.69 ± 6.51	[0.06; 5.32]	16.06	0.06 *
3 [W]	39.23 ± 23.01	34.81 ± 21.14	4.42 ± 8.64	[0.93; 7.91]	22.08	0.02 *
4 [P]	45.38 ± 25.57	40.19 ± 20.02	5.19 ± 18.35	[−2.22; 12.60]	23.03	0.16
6 [W]	52.90 ± 28.36	49.04 ± 27.24	3.85 ± 18.12	[−3.47; 11.17]	27.80	0.31
8 [W]	57.86 ± 33.11	55.7 ± 29.86	2.11 ± 16.44	[−4.53; 8.76]	31.54	0.49

* $p < 0.05$; [P] = paired *t*-test; [W] =Wilcoxon signed-rank test; G: more glaucomatous eyes or more affected glaucomatous eyes; NG: non glaucomatous eyes or less affected glaucomatous eyes; CI: confidence interval.

3.4. Paired t-Tests for Speech Frequencies

The differences in combined speech frequencies (0.5, 0.7, 1, 1.5, 2, 3, and 4 kHz) between ears corresponding to glaucomatous or more affected glaucomatous eyes and contralateral ears were evaluated [11]. Given that the combined speech frequencies for ears corresponding to non-glaucomatous or less glaucomatous eyes did not follow a normal distribution (Shapiro–Wilk $p = 0.042$), the Wilcoxon signed-rank test was used. The test results of this non-parametric test indicated a statistically significant difference in the combined speech frequencies between the ears corresponding to the glaucomatous or more affected glaucomatous eyes and the contralateral ears ($p = 0.022$). The mean difference in hearing thresholds was 2.40 dB, with a bootstrapped 95% confidence interval ranging from 0.67 to 4.13 dB. Despite the effect size (Cohen's d = 0.21) indicating a modest clinical impact, these findings imply that glaucoma may still affect auditory function, particularly across these combined speech frequencies. This supports the hypothesis that patients with unilateral or more severe glaucoma could experience worse hearing in the ear corresponding to the glaucomatous or more affected eye.

3.5. Correlation Analysis

The correlation analysis between RNFL and MD values for glaucomatous or more affected glaucomatous eyes and PTA of the corresponding ears was performed. The Shapiro–Wilk Test for normality indicated that most PTA values were normally distributed

(p-value > 0.05), allowing for Pearson's correlation analysis, except for PTA at 0.125 and 6 kHz frequencies and g-RNFL for glaucomatous eyes (p-value $\leq$ 0.05), thus requiring Spearman's correlation analysis.

3.5.1. Normality Testing

The Shapiro–Wilk Test for normality indicated that most PTA values were normally distributed (p-value > 0.05), allowing for Pearson's correlation analysis, except for PTA at 0.125 and 6 kHz frequencies and g-RNFL for glaucomatous eyes (p-value $\leq$ 0.05), thus requiring Spearman's correlation analysis.

3.5.2. RNFL and PTA

Pearson's correlation coefficients ranged from −0.21 to 0.04, indicating very weak correlations (mostly negative) between PTA values at various frequencies and RNFL. Spearman's correlation coefficients at non-normally distributed frequencies also showed very weak correlations. None of the p-values were below 0.05, indicating that none of these correlations are statistically significant.

3.5.3. MD and PTA

Pearson's correlation coefficients ranged from −0.19 to −0.38, indicating weak to moderate negative correlations between PTA values at various frequencies and MD of glaucomatous or more affected eyes. The closest to statistical significance was at 4 kHz (p = 0.0568).

Although the Pearson and the Spearman correlation analyses between RNFL and PTA values were weak, the negative direction of most correlations suggests a potential trend where thinner RNFL may be associated with worse hearing thresholds. Similarly, the Pearson correlation coefficients between MD values and PTA ranged from −0.12 to −0.38, indicating weak to moderate negative correlations. These negative correlations imply that as the severity of visual field loss (as measured by MD) increases, hearing thresholds tend to worsen. The correlation at 4 kHz was the closest to significance (p-value = 0.0568), suggesting a potential trend that warrants further investigation.

3.5.4. Difference Analysis

The results of the correlation analysis are detailed in Table 3. The correlation analysis between the difference in RNFL and MD values for glaucomatous or more affected glaucomatous eyes and the difference in PTA of the corresponding ears was performed. The correlation between differences in MD and PTA at 0.125 kHz showed a moderately positive correlation, with a Pearson's correlation coefficient equal to 0.5002284 (p = 0.009). The correlations generally show that as the difference in PTA between ears corresponding to glaucomatous and non-glaucomatous eyes increases, there tends to be a corresponding increase in the difference in MD values, thus implying that the degree of hearing loss in the ear corresponding to the glaucomatous eye may be related to the severity of visual field loss. However, the strength of these correlations varies across different frequencies, with some frequencies showing moderate positive correlations (e.g., PTA 0.125 and PTA 8), while others show weaker correlations or no correlation at all (e.g., PTA 1, PTA 3, PTA 4). The correlation between differences in RNFL and PTA at 0.125 kHz showed a moderately positive correlation (r = 0.373; p = 0.06), indicating that as PTA differences increase, RNFL differences tend to increase moderately, while the correlation between differences in RNFL and PTA at the other frequencies were weak, suggesting that this relationship may be more pronounced at lower frequencies. The results of the difference analysis are detailed in Table 4.

Table 3. Correlation analysis between RNFL and PTA and MD and PTA at the studied frequencies.

PTA Frequency (kHz)	RNFL and PTA		MD and PTA	
	Pearson's Correlation Coefficient	*p*-Value	Pearson's Correlation Coefficient	*p*-Value
0.125	0.08	0.71	−0.23	0.26
0.250	−0.17	0.40	−0.19	0.34
0.5	−0.12	0.56	−0.22	0.27
0.7	−0.17	0.43	−0.34	0.10
1	−0.11	0.58	−0.30	0.13
1.5	−0.11	0.59	−0.28	0.19
2	−0.21	0.30	−0.34	0.09
3	−0.17	0.40	−0.32	0.10
4	−0.17	0.40	−0.38	0.06
6	−0.02	0.90	−0.32	0.11
8	0.04	0.85	−0.28	0.16

Table 4. Correlation analysis between difference in RNFL and difference in PTA; difference in MD and difference in PTA at the studied frequencies. Δ: difference.

PTA Frequency (kHz)	ΔRNFL and ΔPTA		ΔMD and ΔPTA	
	Pearson's Correlation Coefficient	*p*-Value	Pearson's Correlation Coefficient	*p*-Value
0.125	0.37	0.06	0.50	0.01
0.250	−0.11	0.59	0.23	0.25
0.5	−0.13	0.54	0.24	0.24
0.7	0.03	0.90	0.27	0.21
1	−0.06	0.77	0.13	0.51
1.5	−0.01	0.96	0.18	0.41
2	0.06	0.76	0.23	0.26
3	−0.36	0.07	-0.03	0.89
4	−0.24	0.24	0.03	0.89
6	−0.27	0.18	0.10	0.64
8	−0.07	0.73	0.30	0.14

4. Discussion

The present study explores the potential link between unilateral or asymmetric glaucoma and ipsilateral hearing impairment, with a specific focus on correlations between RNFL thickness, visual field MD values, and PTA measurements at various frequencies. Our findings underscore the importance of integrated sensory assessments in the comprehensive management of glaucoma patients, given the emerging evidence of a relationship between ophthalmic and auditory health.

In our study, the correlation analysis between MD and PTA values suggested a moderate negative correlation, implying that as the severity of visual field loss increases, hearing thresholds tend to worsen. Furthermore, the correlation between differences in MD and PTA exhibited a moderate positive correlation, indicating that as the difference in PTA between the glaucomatous and non-glaucomatous eyes increases, there tends to be a corresponding increase in the difference in MD values. This finding suggests that the degree of hearing loss in the ear corresponding to the glaucomatous eye may be related to the severity of visual field loss, particularly at lower (0.125 kHz) and higher (8 kHz) frequencies.

These findings corroborate the observations made by Neacsu et al., who examined the relationship between MD and PTA and identified an indirect association between visual field examination parameters and audiometry results [12].

The analysis revealed a moderately positive correlation between differences in RNFL thickness and PTA values at the 0.125 kHz frequency. This suggests that as the difference in hearing thresholds between the glaucomatous and non-glaucomatous ears increases, the corresponding difference in RNFL thickness tends to increase moderately. This finding implies that the relationship between ophthalmic and auditory parameters may be more pronounced at lower sound frequencies. This observation corroborates the previous finding that linked the difference in MD to the difference in PTA at 0.125 kHz, further underscoring the importance of examining lower frequencies when investigating the potential connection between glaucoma and hearing impairment.

In this we observed statistically significant differences in speech-relevant frequencies—specifically at 0.7, 1, 1.5, and 3 kHz—between ears corresponding to glaucomatous or more affected glaucomatous eyes and their contralateral ears. This suggests that glaucoma may particularly impact auditory function at these speech-relevant frequencies, which could have profound implications for patient's quality of life. The paired *t*-tests and Wilcoxon's signed-rank tests confirmed the statistical significance of these differences, further supporting the hypothesis of a frequency-specific auditory deficit associated with glaucoma. The central, speech-related frequencies appear to be more correlated with glaucoma, potentially because presbycusis typically affects higher frequencies [13]. This age-related HL might reduce the observable difference in hearing thresholds between both sides at higher frequencies. The central frequencies are critical for speech comprehension, and deficits in these ranges can severely impact social interactions and communication. Consequently, the identification of HL at these frequencies underscores the importance of considering hearing rehabilitation options, such as hearing aids, to improve patient's QoL [14].

Hearing impairments primarily impact social functioning, as hearing is crucial for understanding and participating in conversations, which are central to everyday social interactions. In contrast, vision impairment predominantly affects a person's ability to navigate and interact with their physical and spatial environment [10]. Research has shown that individuals with both vision and hearing impairments experience more significant declines in physical and mental health, as evidenced by lower scores on health-related quality of life surveys compared to those with only vision or hearing impairment. This compounded effect occurs because vision and hearing influence different aspects of life, and losing both senses results in a greater overall negative impact than losing either one alone [10]. Moreover, glaucoma itself can significantly impact a patient's QoL in several ways. First, simply receiving a diagnosis of this chronic, irreversible, and potentially blinding disease can cause anxiety and negatively affect well-being [15]. Second, the progressive vision loss associated with glaucoma can lead to difficulties in daily life, affecting activities like reading, driving, and even recognizing faces. This can lead to a loss of independence and social isolation. Finally, the burden of treatment, including the side effects of medications, the inconvenience of drop regimens, and the potential need for surgery, can also negatively impact QoL [15].

The identification of specific frequencies where glaucoma more significantly appears to impact hearing thresholds suggests several broader implications. These findings could influence clinical practices by prompting more comprehensive audiometric evaluations in patients with glaucoma, focusing on the frequencies critical for speech comprehension and communication. This could lead to earlier detection and the management of hearing impairment in this patient population, potentially improving patients' quality of life through timely interventions such as hearing aids. Furthermore, the pronounced impact of glaucoma on hearing at these speech-relevant frequencies suggests a need to explore potential shared mechanisms or pathways between ocular and auditory health, such as vascular or neurodegenerative processes [6–8,16]. Understanding these connections could provide valuable insights into the systemic effects of glaucoma and guide future research and treatment strategies.

The observed association between glaucoma and hearing impairment underscores the need for a holistic approach to patient management. Clinicians should consider routine auditory evaluations in glaucoma patients to identify and address concurrent hearing loss, which can significantly impact patients' daily functioning and social interactions; a multidisciplinary approach involving ophthalmologists and audiologists could enhance patient care, addressing both aspects of sensory impairment.

The primary limitation of this study was its small sample size. Further research with larger participant groups is necessary to confirm the observed trends and could also help to clarify which specific sound frequencies are most affected by the presence of glaucoma. Another limitation of our study was the lack of assessment of patient's QoL through the use of specific questionnaires. The retrospective nature of the study precludes causal inferences. Longitudinal studies are necessary to establish the temporal relationship between glaucoma progression and auditory decline. Additionally, larger studies could help elucidate the underlying mechanisms linking visual and hearing impairments in this condition. Although we applied strict inclusion and exclusion criteria, potential confounders such as systemic diseases (e.g., diabetes, hypertension) could influence the results. Future research should aim to control for these variables to isolate the specific impact of glaucoma on hearing function. Future studies should aim to uncover the mechanisms connecting glaucoma with auditory impairment, particularly at the specific frequencies identified in this research. A deeper understanding of these mechanisms could provide valuable insights into the pathophysiology of glaucoma and its broader systemic effects. Exploring the clinical implications of these findings could lead to more comprehensive management strategies, addressing both visual and auditory health for patients with glaucoma.

5. Conclusions

This study highlights a potential association between unilateral or asymmetric glaucoma and ipsilateral hearing impairment, particularly at specific speech-relevant frequencies. The findings emphasize the importance of integrated sensory assessments in the management of glaucoma patients, with implications for improving overall QoL through early detection and intervention for concurrent HL. Such research has the potential to lead to improved diagnostic and therapeutic approaches, ultimately enhancing the quality of life for individuals with glaucoma by comprehensively addressing both their visual and auditory needs.

Author Contributions: G.M. conceived the original idea of the study; L.A.M. and G.M. designed the study; L.A.M. and M.B. performed the ophthalmology assessment; B.F. and G.V. performed the otorhinolaryngology assessment; L.A.M. wrote the original draft; L.A.M. and G.C. analyzed the data; G.C., G.M., and B.F. reviewed and edited the draft; G.M. and S.D.G. supervised the project. All authors have read and agreed to the published version of the manuscript.

Funding: This research received no external funding.

Institutional Review Board Statement: The study was conducted in accordance with the Declaration of Helsinki and approved by the "Ethic Committee of the University of Rome Tor Vergata, Comitato Etico Territoriale Lazio Area 2"; ethics approval code: R.S. 263.24; ethics approval date: 10 July 2024.

Informed Consent Statement: Informed consent was obtained from all subjects involved in the study.

Data Availability Statement: Data supporting the results are available upon request.

Conflicts of Interest: The authors declare no conflicts of interest.

References

1. Jutley, G.; Luk, S.M.; Dehabadi, M.H.; Cordeiro, M.F. Management of glaucoma as a neurodegenerative disease. *Neurodegener. Dis. Manag.* **2017**, *7*, 157–172. [CrossRef] [PubMed]
2. Meliante, L.A.; Piccotti, G.; Tanga, L.; Giammaria, S.; Manni, G.; Coco, G. Glaucoma, Pseudoexfoliation and Hearing Loss: A Systematic Literature Review. *J. Clin. Med.* **2024**, *13*, 1379. [CrossRef] [PubMed]
3. Vidal-Sanz, M.; Salinas-Navarro, M.; Nadal-Nicolás, F.M.; Alarcón-Martínez, L.; Valiente-Soriano, F.J.; de Imperial, J.M.; Avilés-Trigueros, M.; Agudo-Barriuso, M.; Villegas-Pérez, M.P. Understanding glaucomatous damage: Anatomical and functional data from ocular hypertensive rodent retinas. *Prog. Retin. Eye Res.* **2012**, *31*, 1–27. [CrossRef] [PubMed]
4. Almasieh, M.; Wilson, A.M.; Morquette, B.; Cueva Vargas, J.L.; Di Polo, A. The molecular basis of retinal ganglion cell death in glaucoma. *Prog. Retin. Eye Res.* **2012**, *31*, 152–181. [CrossRef] [PubMed]
5. Coleman, A.L.; Kodjebacheva, G. Risk Factors for Glaucoma Needing More Attention. *Open Ophthalmol. J.* **2009**, *3*, 38–42. [CrossRef] [PubMed]
6. Shoeb Ahmad, S.; Ahmad, S.S. Controversies in the vascular theory of glaucomatous optic nerve degeneration. *Taiwan J. Ophthalmol.* **2016**, *6*, 182–186. Available online: https://www.researchgate.net/publication/305810165_Controversies_in_the_vascular_theory_of_glaucomatous_optic_nerve_degeneration (accessed on 17 December 2023). [CrossRef] [PubMed]
7. Wareham, L.K.; Calkins, D.J. The Neurovascular Unit in Glaucomatous Neurodegeneration. *Front. Cell Dev. Biol.* **2020**, *8*, 552297. [CrossRef] [PubMed]
8. Shi, X. Physiopathology of the cochlear microcirculation. *Hear Res.* **2011**, *282*, 10–24. [CrossRef] [PubMed]
9. Shi, X. Pathophysiology of the cochlear intrastrial fluid-blood barrier (review). *Hear Res.* **2016**, *338*, 52–63. [CrossRef] [PubMed]
10. Chia, E.-M.; Mitchell, P.; Rochtchina, E.; Foran, S.; Golding, M.; Wang, J.J. Association Between Vision and Hearing Impairments and Their Combined Effects on Quality of Life. *Arch. Ophthalmol.* **2006**, *124*, 1465–1470. [CrossRef] [PubMed]
11. Wang, J.; Wang, F.; Han, P.; Liu, Y.; Ma, W.; Zhang, H.; Yu, X.; Xie, F.; Niu, S.; Hu, H.; et al. Gender-specific associations of speech-frequency hearing loss, high-frequency hearing loss, and cognitive impairment among older community dwellers in China. *Aging Clin. Exp. Res.* **1990**, *34*, 857–868. [CrossRef] [PubMed]
12. Neacșu, A.M.; Anton, N.; Lăpușneanu, L.; Mușat, O.; Andrei, M.C.; Coșman, M.; Țovănac, N.A.; Ferechide, D. Dynamics of the association between visual and auditory functional changes in glaucoma. Preliminary results. *Rom. J. Ophthalmol.* **2023**, *67*, 117–127. [CrossRef] [PubMed]
13. Cheslock, M.; De Jesus, O. Presbycusis. *StatPearls [Internet]*. Published Online 23 August 2023. Available online: https://www.ncbi.nlm.nih.gov/books/NBK559220/ (accessed on 1 August 2024).
14. Salmon, M.K.; Brant, J.; Hohman, M.H.; Leibowitz, D. Audiogram Interpretation. In *StatPearls [Internet]*; StatPearls Publishing: Treasure Island, FL, USA, 2024. Available online: https://www.ncbi.nlm.nih.gov/books/NBK578179/ (accessed on 22 October 2024).
15. Quaranta, L.; Riva, I.; Gerardi, C.; Oddone, F.; Floriano, I.; Konstas, A.G.P. Quality of Life in Glaucoma: A Review of the Literature. *Adv. Ther.* **2016**, *33*, 959–981. [CrossRef] [PubMed]
16. Wongrakpanich, S.; Petchlorlian, A.; Rosenzweig, A. Sensorineural organs dysfunction and cognitive decline: A review article. *Aging Dis.* **2016**, *7*, 763–769. [CrossRef] [PubMed]

MDPI AG
Grosspeteranlage 5
4052 Basel
Switzerland
Tel.: +41 61 683 77 34

Journal of Clinical Medicine Editorial Office
E-mail: jcm@mdpi.com
www.mdpi.com/journal/jcm